Rad...

STEVE FORSHIER

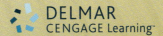

DELMAR
CENGAGE Learning

Australia • Brazil • Japan • Korea • Mexico • Singapore • Spain • United Kingdom • United States

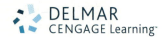

Essentials of Radiation Biology and Protection, Second Edition
Steve Forshier

Vice President, Career and Professional Editorial: Dave Garza

Director of Learning Solutions: Matthew Kane

Senior Acquisitions Editor: Sherry Dickinson

Managing Editor: Marah Bellegarde

Product Manager: Natalie Pashoukos

Editorial Assistant: Jennifer Waters

Vice President, Career and Professional Marketing: Jennifer McAvey

Marketing Director: Wendy Mapstone

Marketing Manager: Michelle McTighe

Marketing Coordinator: Chelsey Iaquinta

Production Director: Carolyn Miller

Production Manager: Andrew Crouth

Content Project Manager: Anne Sherman

Senior Art Director: Jack Pendleton

Technology Project Manager: Christopher Catalina

Production Technology Analyst: Thomas Stover

For product information and technology assistance, contact us at
Professional & Career Group Customer Support, 1-800-648-7450

For permission to use material from this text or product, submit all requests online at **cengage.com/permissions.** Further permissions questions can be e-mailed to **permissionrequest@cengage.com.**

Library of Congress Control Number: 2008925672

ISBN-13: 978-1428312173

ISBN-10: 142831217X

Delmar
5 Maxwell Drive
Clifton Park, NY 12065-2919
USA

Cengage Learning products are represented in Canada by Nelson Education, Ltd.

For your lifelong learning solutions, visit **delmar.cengage.com**

Visit our corporate website at **cengage.com.**

Notice to the Reader

Publisher does not warrant or guarantee any of the products described herein or perform any independent analysis in connection with any of the product information contained herein. Publisher does not assume, and expressly disclaims, any obligation to obtain and include information other than that provided to it by the manufacturer. The reader is expressly warned to consider and adopt all safety precautions that might be indicated by the activities described herein and to avoid all potential hazards. By following the instructions contained herein, the reader willingly assumes all risks in connection with such instructions. The publisher makes no representations or warranties of any kind, including but not limited to, the warranties of fitness for particular purpose or merchantability, nor are any such representations implied with respect to the material set forth herein, and the publisher takes no responsibility with respect to such material. The publisher shall not be liable for any special, consequential, or exemplary damages resulting, in whole or part, from the readers' use of, or reliance upon, this material.

Printed in Canada
1 2 3 4 5 XX 10 09 08

Contents

Preface

INTRODUCTION

Welcome to the second edition of *Essentials of Radiation Biology and Protection*.

Having undergone a thorough update and revision, *Essentials of Radiation Biology and Protection* is designed to provide radiography students with vital information about the biological effects of ionizing radiation and radiation protection to help ensure safe use in diagnostic imaging. This text will assist students in preparation for the American Registry of Radiologic Technologists (ARRT) certification exam. It will also serve as a valuable reference for the practicing radiographer, radiology residents, radiologists, and medical physicists.

It remains vital that we view clinical knowledge and practices as being equally important as theoretical knowledge. This text serves to integrate the theory of radiation protection as seen in radiobiology with radiation protection as it should be practiced in the clinical education setting. Therefore, information presented to the student is both applied and practical.

CONTENT AND ORGANIZATION

Each chapter begins with an outline, objectives, and key terms, and ends with key concepts, review questions, case studies, and Web exercises. The overall text design groups seven chapters into three sections titled: Theory and Concepts, Biological Effects of Radiation Exposure, and Radiation Protection.

Although the ordering of the chapters is based on my experience as a radiography educator, chapters can stand alone, and can be used in the order that is most appropriate within a given program.

Content reflects the most current ARRT Content Specifications for the Examination in Radiography, and American Society of Radiologic Technologists (ASRT) Curriculum Guide.

NEW TO THIS EDITION

In keeping with current trends, updated information has been included that addresses:

- National Council on Radiation Protection (NRCP) recommendations
- Image receptors—digital vs. film
- Pulsed fluoroscopy
- Dosimeters

At the conclusion of each chapter, information is provided that links the chapter contents to the ASRT Curriculum Guide. The ASRT Curriculum Guide is divided into specific content areas. For this text, these content areas include: radiation biology (found in the Guide on pages 54–57) and radiation protection (on pages 61–64). The links provided at the end of each chapter can be found within these respective content areas.

Numerous illustrations and photographs have been added to complement new, updated, or expanded material. Tables have been updated to reflect the most current trends and data.

The student workbook has been integrated into the text to make it a user-friendly worktext. End-of-chapter activities such as crossword puzzles, matching exercises, and multiple choice questions offer students opportunities to test their knowledge of key terms and core concepts.

Each section also contains a practice exam to further aid students in the comprehension of critical topics in the field of radiography.

INSTRUCTOR'S RESOURCES

An Electronic Classroom Manager (ECM) has been created for the instructor. It includes:

- PowerPoint slides
- Computerized test bank
- Image library
- Animations
- Instructor's manual

Approximately 130 PowerPoint slides are available to assist with classroom presentations.

The test bank contains over 250 questions (and answers) in ARRT multiple choice format and Situational Judgment Test (SJT) questions. The test bank is in Exam View Pro software, which allows the instructor to mix and match questions to customize a printable test form, as well as to modify questions or add their own questions to the test bank.

The image library provides approximately 75 illustrations from the text.

Animations on mitosis, meiosis, target theory, and ionizing radiation are included.

The instructor's manual contains an objectives list and lecture outlines for each chapter. Answers to the chapter review questions and exercises, case studies, and section review questions are provided. Worksheets that the instructor can hand out in the classroom and additional learning activities are also included. A list of Internet resources appears at the end of the instructor's manual.

ACKNOWLEDGEMENTS

No text is created without the assistance of many individuals whose names do not appear on the title page. This book is no exception. I would like to express my genuine appreciation and gratitude to the following people who contributed significantly to this project.

First and foremost I wish to express my sincere thanks to Natalie Pashoukos, Cengage Learning Product Manager, for her leadership and enthusiastic support of this text. Natalie kept me motivated and headed in the right direction at all times. I couldn't have done this without her expert guidance.

Thanks to the reviewers for their candid constructive criticism. Their comments and suggestions have been incorporated and have helped to make this edition better than ever.

Appreciation is extended to those who have given permission to reproduce photos, images, illustrations, and diagrams.

I wish to thank the students and instructors who have used this text and given it their overwhelming support.

Last, but certainly not least, my wife Pam, for her understanding and support when I spent evenings and weekends working on this project.

ABOUT THE AUTHOR

Steve Forshier, M.Ed., R.T.(R), has been involved in radiography education for approximately 30 years. He has served as a radiography program director, taught in both the public and private sector, and conducted radiography program accreditation visits. He currently teaches online radiography courses. His hobbies include traveling and golf.

REVIEWERS

Cynthia Smith, MS, RT (R)
Instructor
Monroe Community College
Rochester, NY

Regina Panettieri, MPA, RT (R) (CT)
Adjunct Lecturer/Clinical Instructor
Bronx Community College
Bronx, NY

Barbara Smith, BS, RT (R) (QM) FASRT
Instructor
Portland Community College
Portland, OR

Donna Endicott, M. Ed, RT (R)
Radiography Program Director
Xavier University
Cincinnati, OH

Rex Ameigh, MSLM, BSRT (R)
Director Radiologic Technology Program
Austin Peay State University
Clarksville, TN

Robert Comello M.S., RT, (R) (CDT)
Assistant Professor
Midwestern State University
Wichita Falls, TX

Dawn Couch Moore, M.M.Sc., RT (R)
Assistant Professor and Director
Emory University Medical Imaging Program
Atlanta, GA

Lisa Wood, M.S., RT
Professor/Clinical Coordinator
Salt Lake Community College
West Jordan, UT

Theory and Concepts

Radiobiology may be defined as the branch of science concerned with the methods of interaction and the effects of ionizing radiation on living systems. It is a combination of biology, physics, and epidemiology. Because many radiation effects take place at the cellular level, those people who deal with ionizing radiation should have an understanding of cell structure and function, and how these can be affected by exposure to ionizing radiation. This section focuses on the theory and concepts of radiobiology.

CHAPTER 1

Radiobiology History

KEY TERMS

Direct effect

Epilation

Erythema

Fractionation

Indirect effect

Law of Bergonie and Tribondeau

Mutagenesis

Oxygen effect

Protraction

Rad

Radioactivity

Radiobiology

Rem

Reproductive failure

Roentgen (R)

OBJECTIVES

Upon completion of this chapter, the reader should be able to:

- Discuss the history of radiobiology
- Identify pioneers in the field of radiobiology and their contributions to research
- Define terms related to radiation measurement
- Identify regulations involved with radiobiology

RADIOBIOLOGY HISTORY

Radiobiology is the branch of science concerned with the methods of interaction and the effects of ionizing radiation on living systems. It is a combination of biology, physics, and epidemiology.

The beginning of radiobiology was marked by three significant events:

- Wilhelm Conrad Roentgen's discovery of X-rays in 1895 (Figure 1–1);
- Antoine Henri Becquerel's observance of rays being given off by a uranium-containing substance in 1896 (Figure 1–2); and
- The discovery of radium by Pierre and Marie Curie in 1898.

In the late 1890s, the dean at Vanderbilt University sat for a skull radiograph. His hair fell out three weeks post-exposure. At around this same time, other documented signs and symptoms involving X-rays included cases of skin redness, body part numbness, infection, desquamation, **epilation,** and pain. Possible causes were formulated,

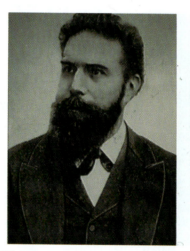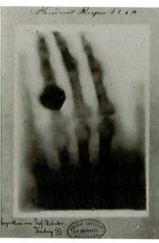

FIGURE 1–1
Wilhelm Conrad Roentgen (Courtesy of the American College of Radiology)

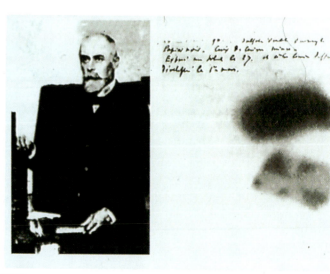

FIGURE 1–2
Becquerel photographic plate (Courtesy of the American College of Radiology)

including ozone production by static machines, excessive heat and moisture, exposure to electricity, and even X-ray allergy. Because there was no historical precedent on which to base a rational fear of X-rays, people had no reason to assume these signs and symptoms could be any more or less damaging than that of electricity.

When viewed against the widespread belief that X-rays were harmless, early questions about radiation safety and efforts at radiation protection became all the more daring. Also in the late 1890s, another radiology pioneer, Elihu Thomson, induced a dermatitis on his finger, and concluded that this was caused by his exposure to X-rays. William Rollins, in his series "Notes on X-Light," emphasized that people should use extreme caution and lead shields when utilizing radiation. Even so, many people disregarded the findings and words of these pioneers, and soon after a variety of zinc lotions and salves were for sale to treat the reddened noses and hands of X-ray personnel.

For many men and women it was already too late. It was not until the death of Clarence Dally (1865–1904), Thomas Edison's assistant in the manufacture of X-ray apparatus, and the documentation of his struggle with burns, serial amputations, and extensive lymph node involvement, that medical observers took seriously the notion that the rays could prove fatal (Figure 1–3).

Due to the lack of proper or complete absence of shielding, Dally was subjected to radiation doses exceeding today's lifetime limits. In Edison's day, protective shielding was seldom used for personnel or X-ray tubes. By 1900, Dally was suffering radiation damage to his hands and face sufficient to require time off work. In 1902, one lesion on his left wrist was treated unsuccessfully with multiple skin grafts and eventually his left hand was amputated. An ulceration on his right hand

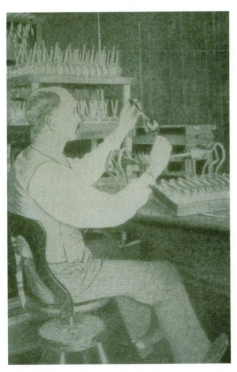

FIGURE 1–3
Clarence Dally (Courtesy of the American College of Radiology)

Notes:

Notes:

necessitated the amputation of four fingers. These procedures failed to halt the progression of his carcinoma, and despite the amputation of his arms at the elbow and shoulder, he died in 1904 from mediastinal cancer. Following this, Thomas Edison abandoned his research on X-rays.

Even then it was difficult to believe in a direct carcinogenic effect from X-rays. Throughout these earliest years, as the obituaries of radiology pioneers appeared with somber regularity in the journals, researchers worked to untangle the paradox by which the new discovery could kill as well as cure.

Early radiologists thought nothing of daily exposure to the rays—to gauge the strength of tubes, perform demonstrations, position and steady patients during therapy, even to calculate an "**erythema** dose" on their own hands. Hand-held fluoroscopy was a common source of exposure in the 1890s (Figure 1–4).

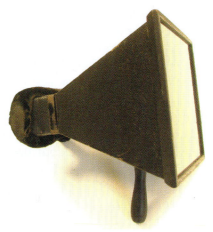

FIGURE 1–4A
Hand-held fluoroscope (Courtesy of Oak Ridge Associated Universities)

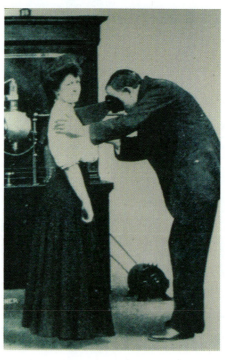

FIGURE 1–4B
Hand-held fluoroscope in use (Courtesy of the American College of Radiology)

This photo shows a roentgenologist seat placed underneath a tilting X-ray table (1898). It provided the radiologist with a comfortable place to sit while performing fluoroscopy, but offered absolutely no protection (Figure 1–5).

Another of the early radiology pioneers, Mihran Kassabian (1870–1910), kept a detailed journal and photographs of his hands while suffering from necroses and subsequent amputations. His intention was that the data he collected would be of importance after his death (Figure 1–6).

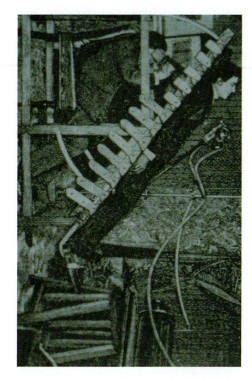

FIGURE 1–5
Roentgenologist seat (Courtesy of the American College of Radiology)

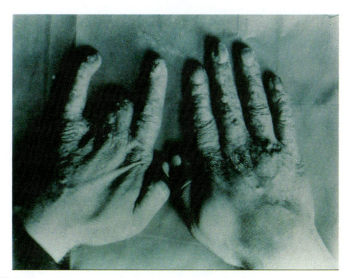

FIGURE 1–6
Mihran Kassabian's hands: necroses and amputations (Courtesy of the American College of Radiology)

Early efforts at protection involved lead screens, heavy aprons, metal helmets, and other paraphernalia, which made the already hot and sometimes noxious practice of radiology even more difficult.

The early observations of Roentgen, Becquerel, the Curies, Edison, and early radiologists sparked research about the effects of radiation exposure on biological processes. From the early 1900s through the 1960s, many theories were developed to define and explain these effects.

Law of Bergonie and Tribondeau

In 1906, radiologist Jean Bergonie and histologist Louis Tribondeau observed the effects of radiation by exposing rodent testicles to X-rays. The testes were selected because they contain both mature and immature cells. The mature cells (spermatozoa) execute the organ's principal function. The immature cells (spermatogonia and spermatocytes) evolve into mature, functional cells. These cells have different cellular functions and their rate of mitosis also differs. The spermatogonia cells divide frequently, whereas the spermatozoa cells do not divide. After irradiating the testes, Bergonie and Tribondeau noticed the immature cells were injured at lower doses than the mature cells. Supported by their observations, they proposed a law describing radiation sensitivity for all body cells. Their law maintains that actively mitotic and undifferentiated cells are most susceptible to damage from ionizing radiation.

The **law of Bergonie and Tribondeau** states that:

1. Stem or immature cells are more radiosensitive than mature cells.
2. Younger tissues and organs are more radiosensitive than older tissues and organs.
3. The higher the metabolic cell activity, the more radiosensitive it is.
4. The greater the proliferation and growth rate for tissues, the greater the radiosensitivity.

This law concludes that compared to a child or mature adult, the fetus is most radiosensitive.

Ancel and Vitemberger

In 1925, embryologists Paul Ancel and P. Vitemberger modified the law of Bergonie and Tribondeau. They suggested that the intrinsic susceptibility of damage to any cell by ionizing radiation is identical, but that the timing of manifestation of radiation-produced damage varies according to the cell type. Their experiments on mammals demonstrated that there are two factors that affect the manifestation of radiation damage to the cell:

1. The amount of biologic stress the cell receives.
2. Pre- and post-irradiation conditions to which the cell is exposed.

Ancel and Vitemberger theorized that the most significant biologic stress on the cell is the need for cell division. They determined that a given dose of radiation will cause the same degree of damage to all cells, but only if and when the cell divides will damage be demonstrated.

Even though Ancel and Vitemberger convey radiosensitivity differently than Bergonie and Tribondeau, they do agree with them by placing a significant emphasis on the amount of mitotic activity involved.

In the 1920s, researchers learned that the process of ionization in tissues was the cause of biologic results. The two mechanisms recognized were:

- Direct ionization along charged particle tracks caused **direct effects** (original ionization occurs directly on target molecule).
- The formation of free radicals caused **indirect effects** (original ionization occurs with water and transfers ionization to target molecule).

Fractionation Theory

In the early days of radiation, it was generally held that the biggest dose (tolerated), given as fast as possible, was the best treatment. During the period, roughly 1920 to 1930, Claude Regaud argued that the differential effect of X-rays on cancer and normal tissues could be best obtained by giving the treatment slowly. For example, healing was very much better when skin cancer was treated over a period of a week than in one day.

Radiologist Regaud exposed sheep testicles to large doses of ionizing radiation. The rams could be sterilized with one large dose, but this quantity of radiation also caused the skin adjacent to the ram's scrotum to have a reaction. It was found that if the original dose was fractionated, or broken up into smaller doses spread out over a period of time, the animals would still become sterile, but with considerably less damage to their skin. Regaud called this the **fractionation theory**.

Repopulation and Protraction

Repopulation primarily refers to the ability of normal tissues to replenish themselves following injury. Because the dose increments are spread out over an extended time, fractionation also involves the element of **protraction**. Protraction is defined as the time during which a course of radiation is given. The logic is that by protracting a course of radiation therapy of five to six weeks, one allows for hyperplastic compensation in some critically affected normal tissues. Although it is likely that no increase in tolerance will be obtained unless the protraction is extended to a period longer than four weeks, some benefit may be obtained from this. The reason for the four-week requirement is that it may take this long for damaged cells to die, to go through the process of lysis, thereby creating a local depletion of cells; and for the remaining cells to mount a replacement proliferation. It is also likely that the tumor cells will continue to proliferate throughout this period.

Mutagenesis

In 1927, geneticist Herman Muller discovered that ionizing radiation produced mutations through his experiments with fruit flies. He found that the radiation-induced mutations were the same as those produced in nature. Irradiating the fruit flies did not create any unusual effects, but the frequency of mutations was intensified. This implies that the effects of ionization were not unique to radiation; that is, they could have been caused by things other than radiation. His finding is termed **mutagenesis**.

Effects of Oxygen and Hydrolysis of Water

The 1940s brought experimentation with oxygen. Geneticist Charles Rick determined oxygen to be a radiosensitizer because it increases the cell-killing effect of a given dose of radiation. This occurs as a result of the increased production of free radicals when ionizing radiation is delivered in the presence of oxygen. This was named the **oxygen effect**.

In 1946 physicist D. Lea did extensive research on the hydrolysis of water with the resulting liberation of free radicals. He termed his finds the mechanism of indirect action.

In 1947, botanists John Read and John Thoday, experimenting with the root tips of *Vicia faba,* discovered that the frequency of chromosome aberrations produced by X-rays depends on the amount of oxygen present during irradiation.

Reproductive Failure

In 1956, geneticists Theodore Puck and Phillip Marcus exposed human uterine cervix cells to varying doses of radiation. They experimentally determined **reproductive failure** by counting the number of colonies formed by these irradiated cells.

In 1959, physicians Mortimer Elkind and H. Sutton-Gilbert, doing cancer research using irradiated Chinese hamster cells, discovered the ability of cells to recover from small radiation doses.

As scientists began to research the effects that radiation exposure had on biological processes, there arose a need to measure the levels of radiation causing specific effects. Units of measurement were developed to quantify radiation levels and thus document the effects of exposure in relation to different levels of exposure.

Roentgen

The term **roentgen** (R) was created in 1928. It was defined as a unit of radiation quantity. The roentgen is a measure of the ionization of air that is created by x- and gamma-radiation below 3 MeV (3 million electron volts). X-ray tube outputs are specified in roentgens or milliroentgens (mR). The adoption of the roentgen as a unit of measurement created the basic tool for defining standards of protection for personnel. In 1937, the roentgen was internationally accepted, and is defined as $1\ R = 2.58 \times 10^{-4}$ coulomb/kg air.

Rad

In 1953, the **rad** (an acronym for radiation absorbed dose) was officially adopted. One rad equals the absorption of 10^{-2} joule (J) of energy per kilogram (or 100 ergs/g) of absorbing material.

$$1 \text{ rad} = 10^{-2} \text{ J/kg} = 100 \text{ ergs/g}$$

The rad describes the energy that is absorbed in matter from any type of ionizing radiation, and is considered the unit of absorbed dose.

Rem

The **rem** (an acronym for radiation equivalent man) is the unit of dose equivalent (DE) or occupational exposure. The rem represents the amount of radiation received by personnel. The rem is said to have approximately the same biologic effectiveness as 1 rad of X-ray. Thus, 1 R = 1 rad = 1 rem in diagnostic radiology.

SI Units

In 1948, the International Committee for Weights and Measures developed a system of measurement that was meant to standardize units of radiation measurement among all professions. This system of measurement is known as the System Internationale d'Unites, or SI units. Within this system of radiation measurement, exposure is measured by coulomb per kilogram and replaces the roentgen. Absorbed dose is expressed by the gray (Gy), which replaces the rad. One gray is equivalent to 100 rads. The equivalent dose is expressed by the sievert, formerly known as the rem. Although the National Council on Radiation Protection and Measurement adopted the use of SI units in 1985, traditional units are still in use. Table 1–1 presents the conversion of traditional units to SI units. Table 1–2 compares both the SI and traditional units.

TABLE 1–1

Conversions between Conventional and SI Units

Conventional Unit (Column A)	Conversion Factor (Column B)	SI Unit (Column C)
roentgen	2.58×10^{-4}	coulomb/kilogram
rad	0.01	gray
rem	0.01	sievert
curie	3.7×10^{10}	becquerel

Column A amount multiplied by Column B equals Column C amount.
Column C amount divided by Column B equals Column A amount.

From Carlton, R., & Adler, A. (2006). *Principles of Radiographic Imaging: An Art and a Science* (4th ed.). Clifton Park, NY: Thomson Delmar Learning.

Notes:

TABLE 1–2

Comparison between SI and Conventional Units

Quantity	Symbol for Quantity	Expression in SI Units	Expression in Symbols for SI Units	Special Name for SI Units	Symbol Using Special Name	Conventional Unit	Symbol for Conventional Unit	Value of Conventional Unit in SI Units
Activity	A	1 per second	s^{-1}	becquerel	Bq	curie	Ci	3.7×10^{10} Bq
Absorbed Dose	D	joule per kilogram	J/kg	gray	Gy	rad	rad	0.01 Gy
Dose Equivalent	H	joule per kilogram	J/kg	sievert	SV	rem	rem	0.01 Sv
Exposure	X	coulomb per kilogram	C/kg	coulomb per kilogram	C/kg	roentgen	R	2.58×10^{-4} C/kg

From Carlton, R., & Adler, A. (2006). *Principles of Radiographic Imaging: An Art and a Science* (4th ed.). Clifton Park, NY: Thomson Delmar Learning.

REGULATION

Many different organizations and agencies are responsible for the development of standards and regulations for radiation protection. These groups include the International Commission of Radiological Protection (ICRP) formed in 1928; and in the United States, the National Council on Radiation Protection and Measurement (NCRP) chartered by Congress in 1964, the Nuclear Regulatory Commission (NRC), and the Food and Drug Administration (FDA).

The International Commission of Radiological Protection (ICRP) and the National Council on Radiation Protection and Measurement (NCRP) first began promoting the idea of regulating the amount of exposure for personnel in the field of radiography in 1931. Based upon the research of these two organizations, the recommended permissible dose was set at 0.2R per day. In 1962, the personnel maximum permissible dose (MPD), now known as effective dose limit, was set at 5 rem per year.

In 1977, the International Council on Radiation Protection (ICRP) Publication 26 set an annual occupational exposure limit of 5 rem per year, and the dose limit for the public of 500 mrem (0.5 rem) per year. In 1991, the ICRP further reduced the occupational exposure limit to 2 rem per year. This recommendation is not yet being enforced in the United States.

In January of 1994, the Nuclear Regulatory Commission (NRC) set effective dose limits based on the National Council on Radiation Protection (NCRP) Report No. 91, which had limits of 5 rem per year for occupational exposure, and 0.1 rem for continuous or frequent exposure per year for the public. The public was allowed 0.5 rem annually for infrequent exposure.

NCRP Report No. 116 is currently used, and supersedes those recommendations contained in NCRP Report No. 91. Report No. 116 still uses the limits of 5 rem per year for occupational exposure; and for the general public, 0.1 rem for continuous or frequent exposure per year, and 0.5 rem for infrequent exposure.

KEY CONCEPTS

- Wilhelm Conrad Roentgen is credited with founding the field of radiobiology with his discovery of X-rays. Much research was done in the 1920s on the effects of radiation on biological processes. Today research continues on the effects of low-level radiation in exposed workers.

- Bergonie and Tribondeau theorized that younger, immature tissues and organs are more radiosensitive than older tissues and organs. They also discovered that as the metabolic activity increases within a cell, the more radiosensitive the cell was. Ancel and Vitemberger determined that radiation damage is determined by the amount of biological stress the cell receives and the conditions the cell is exposed to before and after radiation. Muller made the discovery of radiation's role in mutation, termed mutagenesis.

- The roentgen is a unit of radiation quantity (1 R = 2.58×10^{-4} coulomb/kg). Rad measures the energy absorbed in matter from any type of radiation (1 rad = 10^{-2} J/kg = 100 ergs/g). Rem is the unit of dose equivalent or occupational exposure.

- Five rem per year is the effective dose limit for occupational exposure. 0.1 rem is the limit for frequent public exposure, and 0.5 rem is the limit for infrequent public exposure.

Notes:

REVIEW QUESTIONS & EXERCISES

Crossword Puzzle

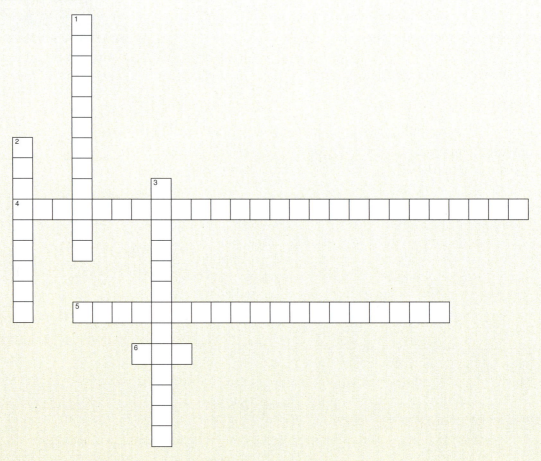

Across

4. States that ionizing radiation is more effective against cells which are highly mitotic, immature, and have a long dividing future.

5. Cell that is unable to continue repeated divisions after being irradiated.

6. The unit of radiation absorbed dose.

Down

1. Division of biology concerned with effects of ionizing radiation on living things.

2. Hair loss.

3. The splitting of radiation into smaller amounts over a period of time.

Matching

Match the definition in the right column with the correct term from the left column.

_____ **1.** Direct effect

_____ **2.** Erythema

_____ **3.** Indirect effect

_____ **4.** Mutagenesis

_____ **5.** Radioactivity

_____ **6.** Rem

_____ **7.** Roentgen

a. The unit of dose equivalent or occupational exposure

b. A result of ionization and excitation, an interaction that happens directly on a critical biologic macromolecule

c. A cell interaction that occurs when the initial ionizing incident takes place on a distant noncritical molecule, which then transfers the ionization of energy to another molecule

d. Reddening of the skin

e. A unit of radiation exposure descriptive of x- or gamma radiation, the quantity of which would produce a charge

f. The capability of a material to give off rays or particles from its nucleus

g. The causing of genetic mutation by radiation

Multiple Choice

1. The Law of Bergonie and Tribondeau states:
   a. that stem cells are more radiosensitive than mature cells.
   b. that older tissues and organs are more radiosensitive than younger tissues and organs.
   c. that the lower the metabolic activity of a cell, the more radiosensitive it is.
   d. the lower the proliferation and growth rate for tissues, the lower the radiosensitivity.

2. The _____ is the unit of dose equivalent or occupational exposure.
   a. roentgen (R)   c. rad
   b. rem   d. erythema

3. Which of the following would be considered most radiosensitive?
   a. fetus   c. teenage patient
   b. pediatric patient d. adult patient

4. The unit of radiation quantity is the _____.
   a. rem   c. roentgen
   b. rad   d. curie

5. Which researcher discovered mutations related to exposure to ionizing radiation?
   a. Muller   c. Roentgen
   b. Becquerel   d. Curie

6. Radiation-induced skin reddening is the definition of:
   a. epilation   c. erythema
   b. anemia   d. radioactivity

7. Which researcher died due to the cumulative effects of radiation?
   a. Wilhelm Roentgen c. Marie Curie
   b. Thomas Edison   d. Clarence Dally

EXPLORING THE WEB

1. Search the Web for additional information on the history of radiobiology. Create a timeline showing the progress made from the early discoveries to today.

    _____

    _____

    _____

    _____

2. Search the Web for current research being done in the area of radiobiology. What new discoveries or theories are on the horizon? What impact may these new discoveries have on current practice?

    _____

    _____

    _____

    _____

3. Search the Web for regulations in the field of radiobiology. Find the Web sites of agencies responsible for enforcing and revising regulations. Are there any new regulations pending? What are the penalties for failing to meet regulations? What additional information can you find pertaining to regulation in the field of radiobiology?

    _____

    _____

    _____

    _____

CASE STUDY

A 22-year-old female is scheduled for a barium enema study. As you are taking her patient history, she informs you there is a possibility she might be pregnant. Discuss how the law of Bergonie and Tribondeau could determine the radiologist's decision on whether to perform the exam on your patient.

_____

_____

_____

_____

_____

_____

CHAPTER 2

Cellular Anatomy and Physiology

KEY TERMS

Amino acid

Anabolism

Anaphase

Autosomes

Catabolism

Centromere

Chromatid

Chromatin

Chromosome

Deoxyribonucleic acid (DNA)

Diploid

DNA proofreading

Duplication

Enzyme

G_1

G_2

Gamete

Gene

Haploid

OBJECTIVES

Upon completion of this chapter, the reader should be able to:

- Indicate the parts of the cell
- Identify organic compounds and their functions
- Identify inorganic compounds and their functions
- Explain mitosis
- Explain meiosis

Notes: _____

CELL BIOLOGY

In order to appreciate radiation interactions within cells, a review of cell biology is necessary. All living things, whether plant or animal, are made up of cells. The cell is the basic unit of structure and function of all living things. It is at the cellular level that the fundamental life functions occur. These essential functions include metabolism, growth, irritability, adaptability, repair, and reproduction. All cells are made up of chemical material called **protoplasm**. The cell is the smallest unit of protoplasm capable of existing independently.

Humans contain between 60 and 100 trillion cells. These cells vary in size, shape, and function. With the exception of human ovum or egg cells, human cells are microscopic in size. They are measured in units called micrometers (μm), or microns (μ) (1 μm or μ = $1/1,000,000$ or 0.000001 or 10^{-6} or approximately $1/25,000$ of an inch). These units of measurement are used when describing cell sizes and their cell components (Figure 2–1).

Regarding shape, human cells differ tremendously. Their shapes may be spherical, rectangular, or irregular. The human body has numerous distinct types of cells, each of which is specialized in performing particular functions. Bone cells, muscle cells, fat cells, blood cells, and nerve cells are examples of specialized cells (Figure 2–2). Cell structure is directly related to its function.

Tissues are collections of similar cells that work together in performing a particular function. An example of a tissue is muscle. Muscles function to contract and cause movement of body parts.

An organ is a combination of two or more tissues that are combined to perform a specific function. Organs vary greatly in their size and function. The heart, spleen, and pancreas are examples of organs.

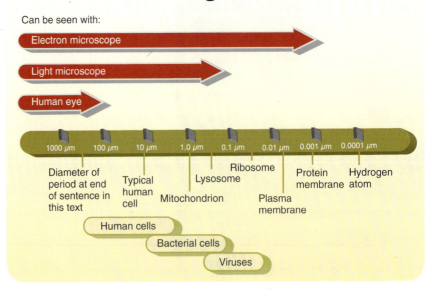

Size Range of Cells

FIGURE 2–1
Cell size

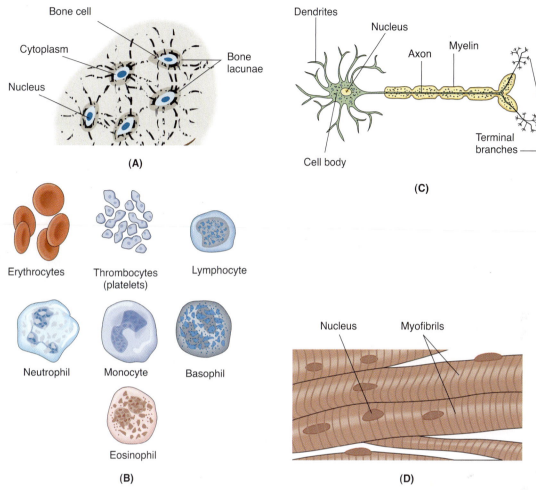

FIGURE 2–2
Human cell types: (A) Bone, (B) Blood, (C) Neuron, (D) Skeletal muscle

The system is the next level of structural organization (Figure 2–3). Organs that have similar or related functions comprise a body system. The digestive system and circulatory system are examples of systems. All the body systems work together and are interrelated to form the total organism.

Chemical Configuration of Cells

Protoplasm contains organic and inorganic compounds. These are either dissolved or suspended in water, which is the most abundant component of protoplasm. Protoplasm contains 70–85% water. The percentage of water in protoplasm depends upon the type of cell. Water makes up approximately 55–75% of a person's total body weight, and for several reasons is essential to life (Figure 2–4).

The critical functions of water in the body include:

• action as a solvent, that is, various substances can dissolve in water
• acts as a transport medium for substances
• serves to lubricate joints and the digestive tract
• regulates body temperature through evaporation
• cushions organs such as the brain and lungs

Notes:

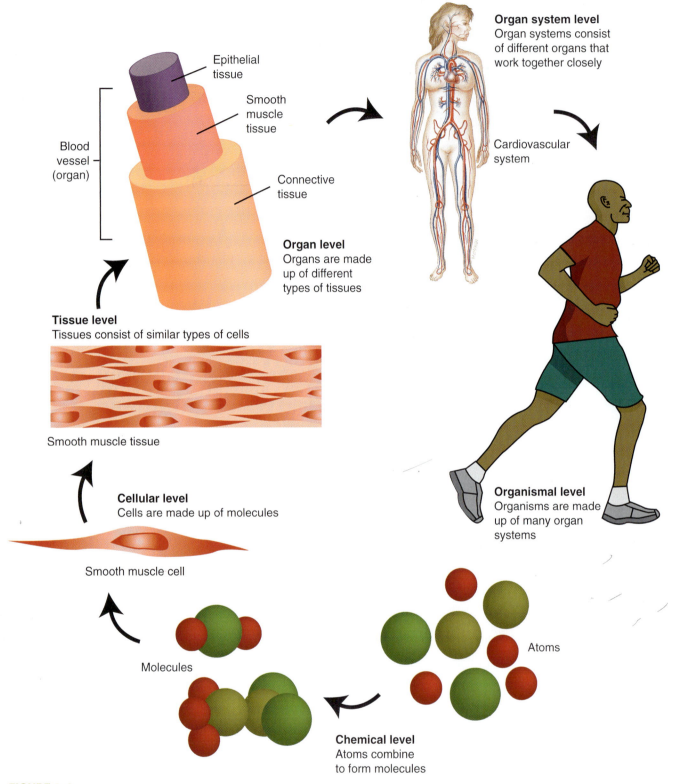

Organ system level
Organ systems consist of different organs that work together closely

Cardiovascular system

Epithelial tissue

Smooth muscle tissue

Blood vessel (organ)

Connective tissue

Organ level
Organs are made up of different types of tissues

Tissue level
Tissues consist of similar types of cells

Smooth muscle tissue

Organismal level
Organisms are made up of many organ systems

Cellular level
Cells are made up of molecules

Smooth muscle cell

Atoms

Molecules

Chemical level
Atoms combine to form molecules

FIGURE 2–3
Levels of structural organization

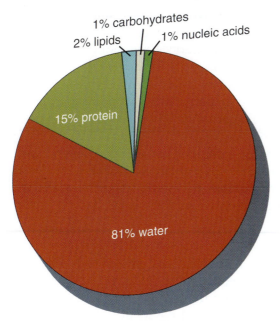

FIGURE 2–4
Chemical configuration of cells

Organic Compounds   Organic compounds denote chemical substances that contain carbon. The four major classes of organic compounds found in cells include proteins, carbohydrates, nucleic acids, and lipids.

Proteins   Proteins, which comprise 15% of the cell, are composed of the elements carbon, hydrogen, oxygen, and nitrogen. Proteins are found in all parts of a living cell. Functions of proteins include: assisting in growth, constructing new tissues, and repairing injured or worn-out tissues. Enormous amounts of proteins are located in fingernails, hair, cartilage, ligaments, tendons, and muscle.

   Amino acids are the building blocks of proteins. In humans there are 22 different amino acids that combine in numerous sequences to create proteins. The number of amino acids in proteins ranges from 300 to several thousand. Examples of proteins include insulin, egg whites, gelatin, and hemoglobin.

   Enzymes are an important group of proteins that are found in all living cells. Enzymes act as organic catalysts. They control the numerous chemical reactions that occur in cells. Enzymes provide cell energy, help to make new cell parts, and control almost every cell process. They affect the rate or speed of chemical reactions without themselves being altered.

Lipids   Lipids comprise approximately 2% of the cell. Lipids contain carbon, hydrogen, and oxygen, and exist in all living cells. Lipids function in storing energy, insulating our bodies from cold, assisting with the digestive process, and helping to lubricate the joints.

Carbohydrates   Carbohydrates make up approximately 1% of the cell. They are composed of carbon, hydrogen, and oxygen, and are the major source of cell energy. Even though carbohydrates are found throughout the body, they are located predominately in the liver and muscles. Carbohydrates are subdivided into monosaccharides, disaccharides, and polysaccharides. Monosaccharides are considered simple sugars. They cannot be broken down further. Examples are glucose, fructose, and galactose. Disaccharides are known as double sugars. Examples include sucrose (table sugar), and lactose (milk sugar). Polysaccharides are large **macromolecules** constructed of hundreds to thousands of simple sugar molecules in a long chain. Examples include starch and cellulose.

Nucleic Acids   Nucleic acids are organic compounds that contain carbon, oxygen, hydrogen, and phosphorus. They are the largest known organic molecules. Nucleic acids are high-molecular-weight **polymers** made from thousands of smaller subunits called nucleotides. Nucleotides are composed of a five-carbon sugar (pentose sugar), a phosphate or phosphoric acid group, and one of many nitrogenous bases. There are two groups of nitrogenous bases, purines and pyrimidines. Purines are either adenine (A) or guanine (G). The pyrimidines are cytosine (C), thymine (T), or uracil (U).

The nucleic acids include **DNA (deoxyribonucleic acid)** and **RNA (ribonucleic acid)**.

Inorganic Compounds   Mineral salts, the inorganic substance in the cell, are essential for cell life. Sodium (Na) and potassium (K) are examples of salts. Potassium inside the cell prevents the cell from collapsing. Sodium outside the cell prevents the cell from bursting. Sodium and potassium maintain the osmotic pressure of the cell by maintaining the correct proportion of water in the cell. Salts are required in order for the cell to function correctly. For example, if there were a deficiency of calcium salts in the cell, muscle cramps would occur. Salts also assist in producing cell energy and in conducting nerve impulses.

Cell Structure

Even though human cells can be very different, they also have many similar structural characteristics: a cell membrane, cytoplasm, and organelles (Figure 2–5).

With the exception of mature red blood cells, all human cells have a nucleus. The cytoplasm, organelles, and nucleus are enclosed by a cell membrane.

Cell Membrane   All human cells are surrounded by cell membranes, sometimes called plasma membranes. A cell membrane functions to separate the cell's interior from its exterior surroundings, and also from adjacent cells (Figure 2–6). Although it is the outer boundary of the cell, a cell membrane is not static, but instead is

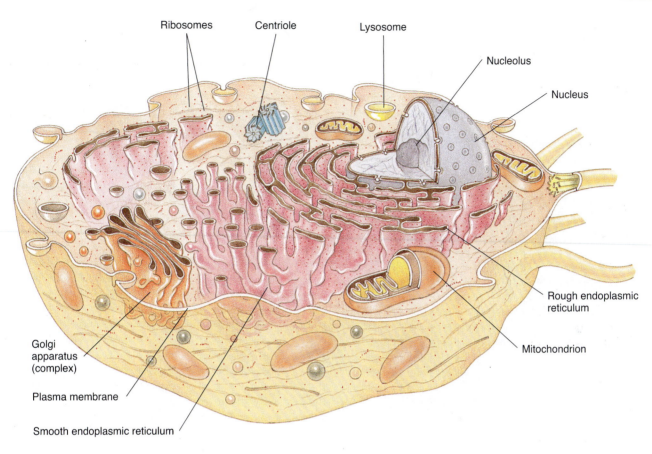

Ribosomes   Centriole   Lysosome

Nucleolus

Nucleus

Rough endoplasmic
reticulum

Mitochondrion

Golgi
apparatus
(complex)

Plasma membrane

Smooth endoplasmic reticulum

FIGURE 2–5
Cell structure

active and dynamic. Cell membranes are composed of lipids and proteins, which are arranged in a double layer somewhat comparable to a sandwich: the two protein layers are the slices of bread and the lipids are the filling.

The cell membrane is considered to be selectively semi-permeable. It allows some substances to pass into and out of the cell, while preventing the passing of others. Lipids allow lipid-soluble materials to diffuse into or out of the cell. Proteins function as pores, enzymes, or antigens.

Cytoplasm   Cytoplasm, composed of proteins, lipids, carbohydrates, minerals, salts, and water, is a watery solution found between the nucleus and cell membrane. Chemical reactions, such as protein synthesis and cellular respiration, take place in the cytoplasm. **Catabolism** (the process of converting a complex substance into a simpler substance) and **anabolism** (the building up of a body's substance) take place in the cytoplasm. Metabolism is the combination of catabolism and anabolism.

Organelles   Cell organelles, located within the cytoplasm, help with cell functioning. Cell organelles include the centrioles, endoplasmic reticulum, mitochondria, Golgi apparatus, lysosomes, and the nucleus.

Notes:

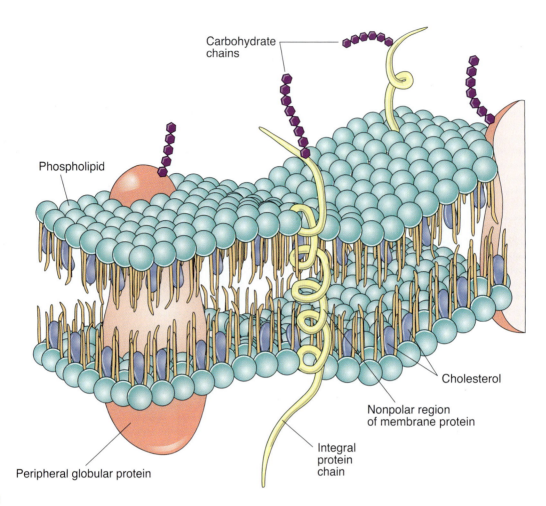

Carbohydrate chains

Phospholipid

Peripheral globular protein

Cholesterol

Nonpolar region of membrane protein

Integral protein chain

FIGURE 2–6
Cell membrane

Notes: _____

The Centrosome and Centrioles   The centrioles, a pair of cylindrical organelles located near the nucleus, are perpendicular to each other, and function to organize the spindle fibers during cell mitosis. They are contained in a circular body named the centrosome. During mitosis, the pair of centrioles detach from each other. During this detachment, thin cytoplasmic spindle fibers are formed between the centrioles. This formation is known as the spindle-fiber apparatus. Spindle fibers connect to specific chromosomes to aid with the equal disbursement of these chromosomes to two daughter cells.

The Endoplasmic Reticulum   The endoplasmic reticulum (ER) is a tubular network that extends from the nuclear membrane to the cell membrane. The endoplasmic reticulum assists in channeling proteins and lipids into and out of the nucleus. Some ER collect copious amounts of proteins and thus serve as storage areas. The two types of ER are rough and smooth. A rough ER has numerous ribosomes attached to its outer surface, giving it a rough appearance. It is found in cells that are active secretors of proteins, such as the endocrine and exocrine glands. A smooth ER has no ribosomes attached to it. It is a site for enzyme reactions in steroid hormone production and inactivation, and is the part of the cell where many drugs are inactivated. It also serves in storing Ca^{++} in skeletal muscle cells.

The Mitochondria   Mitochondria are double-membraned, oval or rod-shaped organelles found in the cytoplasm. The shape and number of mitochondria vary from one cell to another. Aerobic (oxygen-requiring) reactions of cell respiration take place within the mitochondria. The double-membrane of the mitochondria contains enzymes, which assist in breaking down carbohydrates, fat, and proteins into energy, stored in the cell as ATP (adenosine-triphosphate). Cells that require large amounts of ATP contain the greatest amount of mitochondria, such as muscle cells. Because mitochondria supply the cell's energy, they are nicknamed the "powerhouses" of the cell.

The Golgi Apparatus   The Golgi apparatus, also called Golgi bodies or the Golgi complex, was discovered in 1898 by the Italian scientist Camillo Golgi. It is a series of flat, membranous layers, looking somewhat like a stack of pancakes or saucers. Synthesized within the Golgi apparatus are carbohydrates. These carbohydrates are combined with proteins as they pass through the Golgi apparatus, and are concentrated and packaged for secretion from the cell. In order to secrete a substance, small portions of the Golgi membrane separate and join with the cell membrane, which allows the substance to be released to the cell's exterior. These organelles are most abundant in the gastric gland cells, salivary glands, and pancreatic glands.

Lysosomes   Lysosomes are single-membrane oval or spherical bodies within the cytoplasm which contain digestive enzymes that digest protein molecules. Lysosomes assist in digesting old, worn-out cell parts, dead cells, bacteria, and foreign materials. If a lysosome happens to burst, it begins to digest the cell's protein, causing cell death. This is how they acquired the nickname "suicide bags."

The Nucleus   The most vital cell organelle is the nucleus. The nucleus is the brain for the cell's metabolic activity and cell division. Spherical in shape, it is usually located in or near the cell's center. The nucleus floats within the cytoplasm and is surrounded by a double-layered nuclear membrane. DNA (deoxyribonucleic acid) and protein are contained within the nucleus. DNA and protein are arranged in long threads called **chromatin**. When a cell divides, the chromatin contracts into short, rod-like structures called **chromosomes**. Humans normally have 46 total chromosomes, or 23 pairs.

When particular cells reach certain sizes, they may divide into two new cells. If this occurs, the nucleus divides first by undergoing a process called **mitosis**. During mitosis, nuclear substances are distributed to each new nucleus. Next, the cytoplasm divides approximately in half through the development of a new membrane between the two nuclei. It is exclusively during this process of the nucleus dividing that the chromosomes are visible.

Chromosomes contain the human hereditary blueprint—DNA—which passes from one generation of cells to the next.

Notes:

Notes:

The Nuclear Membrane   The **nuclear membrane** is double-layered and has openings through which substances can travel either from the cytoplasm to the nucleus, or from the nucleus to the cytoplasm. The nuclear membrane's outer layer is contiguous with the ER of the cytoplasm, and contains ribosomes. Surrounding the chromatin and nucleoli is the transparent semi-fluid nucleoplasm.

The Nucleolus and Ribosomes   Each nucleus contains at least one nucleolus. The tiny, spherical-shaped **nucleolus** contains ribosomes composed of RNA (ribonucleic acid) and protein. Ribosomes can travel from the cell's nucleus into the cytoplasm. It is there that ribosomes assist in protein synthesis. Ribosomes exist as single units in the cytoplasm, as clusters called polyribosomes, or joined to the walls of the ER.

DNA and RNA   The DNA nucleotide structure is composed of a phosphate group, a deoxyribose sugar, and the nitrogenous bases adenine, thymine, cytosine, and guanine. The RNA nucleotide consists of a phosphate group, ribose sugar, and the nitrogenous bases adenine, cytosine, guanine, and uracil instead of thymine.

The structure of DNA looks like a coiled ladder, as seen in Figure 2–7.

The two strands of nucleotides are labeled a double helix (coil). The sides of the ladder are formed by the alternating phosphate and sugar molecules. The rungs of the ladder are formed by the pairs of

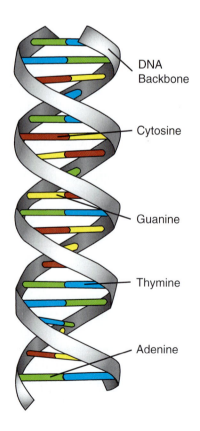

DNA Backbone

Cytosine

Guanine

Thymine

Adenine

FIGURE 2–7
DNA structure

nitrogenous bases. With DNA, adenine always pairs with thymine, and guanine always pairs with cytosine. An acrostic to help you remember these pairings is **A**t **T**he **G**rand **C**anyon. It is estimated that the DNA of our 46 chromosomes includes approximately 6 billion base pairs, which compose 50,000 to 100,000 genes.

Unique genetic information is carried by the DNA located in the nuclear chromosomes and genes. This genetic material instructs the cell as to what structures it will have, and how it will function and behave. The DNA passes genetic information from cell to cell, and ultimately from generation to generation. Thus, DNA is considered the genetic code for heredity characteristics. DNA is located in the plasma membrane, mitochondria, and centrioles.

Instead of being double-stranded like DNA, RNA is a single-stranded nucleotide, with uracil pairing with adenine in place of thymine (Figure 2–8).

RNA is produced from DNA in the cell nucleus, but functions in the cell's cytoplasm.

There are three varieties of RNA. These include **messenger RNA** (m-RNA), **transfer RNA** (t-RNA), and **ribosomal RNA** (r-RNA). Messenger RNA carries directions for protein synthesis from the DNA molecule situated in the cell's nucleus into the cytoplasm, and also carries the code for specific protein synthesis from the DNA in the nucleus to the ribosomes in the cytoplasm. Transfer RNA carries amino acid molecules from the cytoplasm to the ribosomes for protein synthesis. Ribosomal RNA assists in the linking of the messenger RNA to the ribosome. RNA is found in the nucleoli, cytoplasm, and some cell ribosomes.

Chromosomes and Genes   Within the nucleus is the substance responsible for guiding the activity of the cytoplasm. This genetic material is enclosed in chromosomes. Chromosomes are visible only in cells that are dividing. The parts of the chromosome include a **centromere**, which is the center of a chromosome, and arms that extend in each direction from the centromere. (See Figure 2–9.)

The chromosomes carry **genes**, the genetic material responsible for cytoplasmic activity and delivering the cell's hereditary information. Each chromosome contains numerous genes that are situated on the chromosome in a unique linear order. All genes execute specific functions in preserving an organism's life and development.

Sexually reproducing cells in animals are classified as either germ cells or somatic cells. Germ cells are **gametes**: female gametes are termed oocytes and male gametes are called spermatozoa. The somatic cells are all the other cells in the body.

Somatic cells have at least two of each kind of gene situated on two different chromosomes. These two chromosomes are identical in the arrangement and type of genes they carry and are called homologues. Consequently, the chromosomes in somatic cells are paired. Each member of a pair is identical, but the pairs themselves are not alike. The normal number of chromosomes for humans is 46. This number is termed the **diploid** number, or 2n.

Notes:

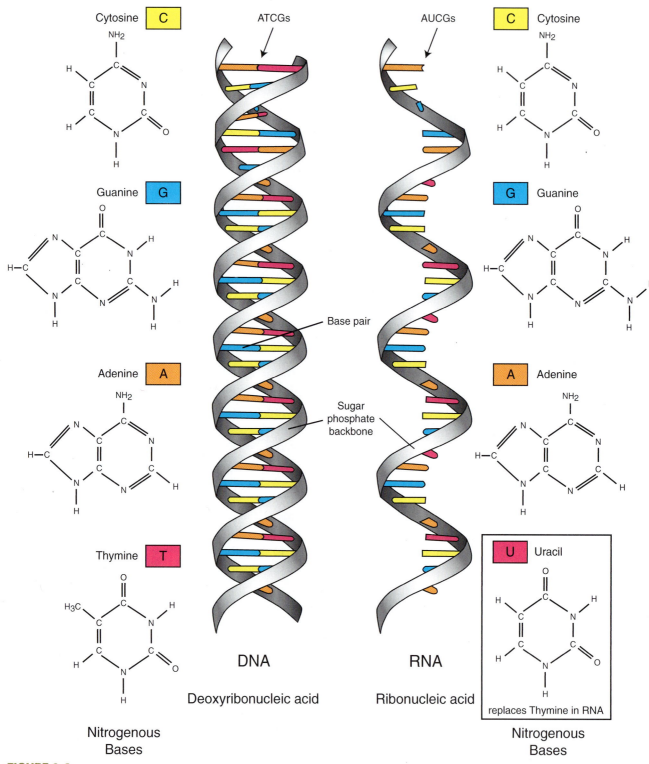

Cytosine C

Guanine G

Adenine A

Thymine T

Nitrogenous
Bases

ATCGs

Base pair

Sugar
phosphate
backbone

DNA
Deoxyribonucleic acid

AUCGs

RNA
Ribonucleic acid

Cytosine C

Guanine G

Adenine A

U Uracil

replaces Thymine in RNA

Nitrogenous
Bases

FIGURE 2–8
DNA vs. RNA structure

Notes:

In germ cells, chromosomes and genes are not paired, but are individual chromosomes. These individual chromosomes come from each of the pairs that exist in the somatic cells. Thus, germ cells contain one-half the number of chromosomes and genes present in somatic cells. The number of chromosomes in germ cells is referred to as the **haploid** or n number.

DNA packs tightly into metaphase chromosomes

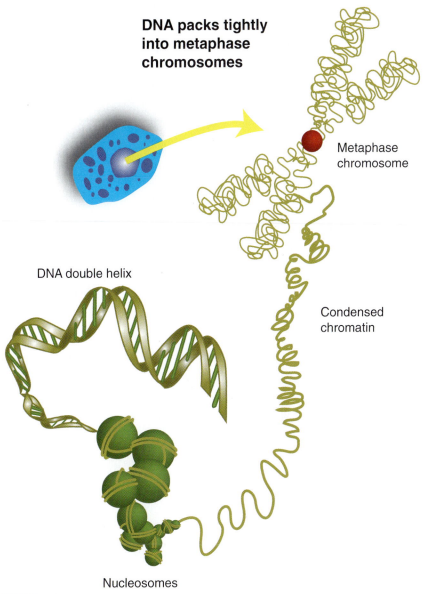

Metaphase chromosome

Condensed chromatin

DNA double helix

Nucleosomes

FIGURE 2–9
DNA metaphase chromosome

In humans, the somatic cells contain 46 chromosomes in the nucleus, of which 44 are **autosomes** (nonsex chromosomes), and 2 are sex chromosomes.

In a human female, somatic cells contain 44 autosomes and 2 sex chromosomes (both are X chromosomes). In the human male, there are also 44 autosomes and 2 sex chromosomes (an X and a Y chromosome).

The human germ cells have one specific function, which is to reproduce the species. During fertilization, the sperm nucleus unites with the egg nucleus to form a fertilized egg, or zygote. Accordingly, it is essential that each germ cell contain only one-half the number of chromosomes to produce a normal zygote that contains the required 2n number of chromosomes (Figure 2–10).

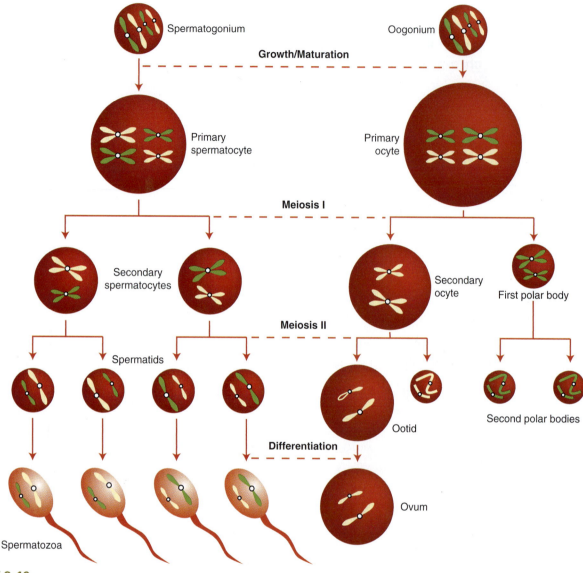

FIGURE 2–10
Gametogenesis

CELL GROWTH AND DIVISION

Cell life follows a cyclical pattern. A new cell is produced as part of its parent cell. When this daughter cell divides, it becomes two new cells. As long as a cell's offspring continue to divide, each cell is conceivably immortal. Some body cells divide constantly; for example, about every two to three days the stomach lining is renewed, and the skin's epidermis is renewed about every two weeks. Conversely, some cells, such as mature nerve cells and skeletal muscle, do not go through division at all.

The two types of cell division are **mitosis** and **meiosis**. Even though both types include reproduction of the cell, their purposes are not similar.

Mitosis

Cell division, or mitosis, can be divided into two discrete processes: the dividing of the nucleus, and the dividing of the cytoplasm.

All human life begins as a fertilized egg. In mitosis, a cell with the diploid number of chromosomes (normally 46) divides into two identical cells, each containing the diploid number of chromosomes. In order for there to be growth of the body and tissue repair, the production of identical cells is essential.

The nondividing cell is in the segment of the cell cycle known as **interphase**, which is subdivided into G_1, S, and G_2. Genes control the metabolism of the cell through their direction of RNA synthesis. Since the cell may be growing during this time, this part of interphase is called the G_1 phase (G = gap or growth). Sometimes referred to as the resting phase, cells in the G_1 phase are performing the physiological purposes necessary to maintaining cell homeostasis. Resting means the cell is not yet undergoing the visible phases of mitosis.

If a cell is to divide, it replicates its DNA in the part of interphase called the **S-phase** (S = synthesis). It is not known what causes transformation of a cell from the G_1 to the S phase (Figure 2–11).

Once there has been replication of DNA, the chromatin condenses into short, thick, rod-like structures. It is in this form that chromosomes are more familiar to us as they can be seen with an ordinary light microscope.

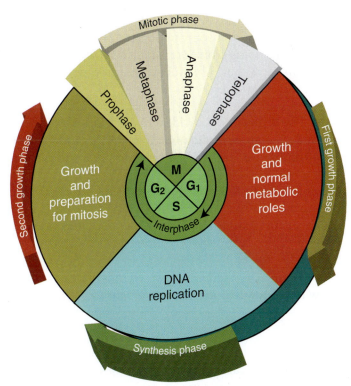

FIGURE 2–11
Cell cycle

Centrosomes are found only in cells that are capable of dividing. During cell division, centrioles position themselves on opposite sides of the nucleus. The centrioles then become involved in the producing of, and are attached to, spindle fibers. During cell division, the centrioles and spindle fibers pull the duplicated chromosomes to opposite poles of the cell. Any cell that lacks centrioles, such as mature nerve and muscle cells, cannot divide. It is during mitosis that cells are the most radiosensitive. The most radioresistant phase of the cell cycle is in late S-phase.

After the S-phase of the cell cycle, each chromosome includes two strands termed chromatids. The chromatids are connected by a centromere. Within a chromosome the two chromatids bear identical DNA base sequences as each is made by DNA replication. Thus, each chromatid contains an entire double helix DNA molecule that is a duplicate of the single DNA molecule that existed before replication. Upon completion of cell division, each chromatid becomes a separate chromosome.

Following G_2, the gap or growth phase following the replication of DNA and prior to mitosis, the cell then enters into the four stages of cell division or mitosis (the M phase of the cell cycle). The stages of mitosis are **prophase**, **metaphase**, **anaphase**, and **telophase**.

Prophase   Chromosomes include two chromatids connected by a centromere. The centrioles migrate toward opposite poles of the cell, producing spindle fibers that extend across the cell's equator. The nuclear membrane begins to disappear, and the nucleolus is no longer visible.

Metaphase   The paired chromosomes are lined up at the equator of the cell. Spindle fibers from each centriole attach to the centromeres of the chromosomes. The nuclear membrane has entirely disappeared and the centromeres now divide.

Anaphase   The centromeres divide and the sister chromatids detach as they are pulled to an opposite pole. Each chromatid is regarded as a separate chromosome, as there are two complete and distinct sets.

Telophase   The sets of chromosomes become much longer, thinner, and indistinct as they reach the poles of the cell. The DNA unravels to form chromatin. There is formation of new nuclear membranes. The nucleolus reappears. Cytokinesis (cell division) is almost complete.

Once the cytoplasm divides, a new cell membrane is constructed and two new daughter cells are formed (Figure 2–12).

Meiosis

In the formation of germ cells, a unique type of cell division transpires in the gonads (ovaries and testes) of sexually mature people. This type of cell division is termed meiosis (Figure 2–13). In the female, the specific meiotic process is labeled oogenesis. In the male, it is called spermatogenesis. Because ova and sperm have one-half

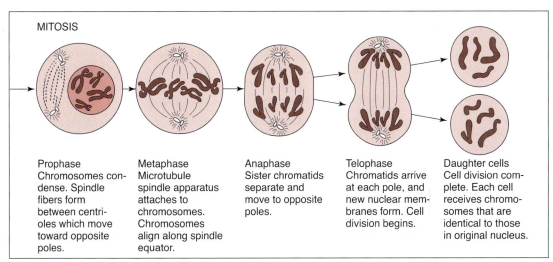

FIGURE 2–12
Mitosis

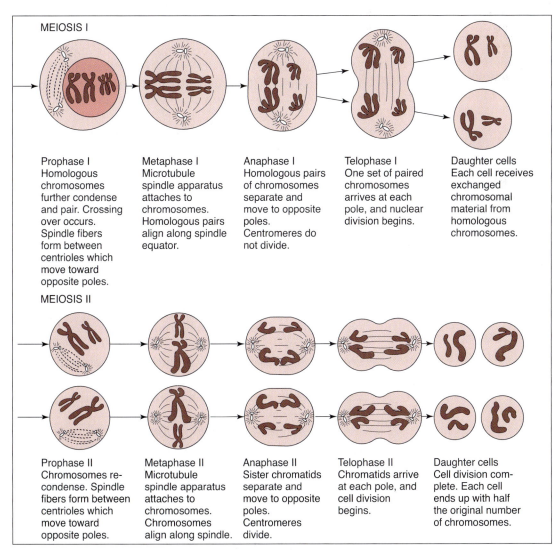

FIGURE 2–13
Meiosis

the number of chromosomes, n (23), as the parent cell, 2n (46), meiosis is also referred to as reduction division. If a zygote is to include the diploid number (2n), it is essential that there is a reduction in the chromosome number of germ cells. If there was not a reduction from 2n to n, this would mean the zygote would acquire two times the required number of chromosomes.

During meiosis, the cell divides twice in succession, but chromosomes are duplicated only once. In both germ and somatic cells, DNA synthesis takes place during interphase, with the result being a **duplication** of each chromosome constructing two chromatids. Thus, at the beginning of meiosis, a germ cell contains twice the amount of genetic material.

The names of the stages for meiosis and mitosis are the same. The movements of the germ cell chromosomes during meiosis are comparable to the way somatic cell chromosomes move during mitosis. At the completion of telophase, the original parent germ cell has created two daughter cells that contain the diploid or 2n (46) number of chromosomes. It is at this moment that the resemblances between meiosis and mitosis end.

The daughter cells then go through a second division of cellular material without replication of the DNA or duplication of the chromosomes. The result of these two successive divisions of meiosis is four gametes, each of which contains the haploid number (23) of chromosomes (Figure 2–14).

DNA Proofreading and Repair

All cells must replicate their DNA prior to cell division. This ensures that each new cell produced receives all of the genetic material necessary to survive and reproduce. As organisms have from thousands to millions or even billions of base-pairs of DNA, this process could seem overwhelmingly complicated. However, cells utilize a relatively simple mechanism to copy their DNA rapidly and accurately. Several different **enzymes** are involved in this process—some unwind the DNA from its double helix, some separate the two strands of DNA, and some build new strands of DNA complementary to each of the original strands. After the DNA is replicated, cells employ several other enzymes to "proofread" their work and correct mistakes from the replication process (Figure 2–15). The result of DNA replication is two complete and accurate copies of a cell's DNA. These copies may then be partitioned into daughter cells during cell division.

It is essential that DNA replication is accurate. Mistakes made during the copying of DNA could completely disrupt important genes, leading to problems or even death for a cell or organism. Fortunately, DNA polymerase does a very accurate job synthesizing new strands of DNA, inserting an incorrect base on average only once in every ten thousand to one million bases. Cells also utilize several other repair processes and enzymes to bring their mistake rate even lower, and ensure that their DNA is replicated accurately.

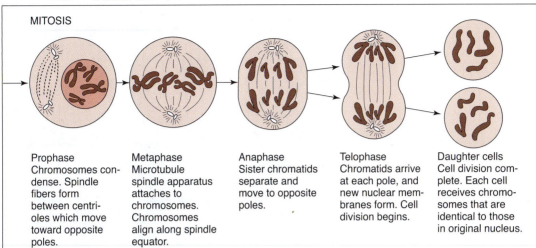

MITOSIS

Prophase
Chromosomes condense. Spindle fibers form between centrioles which move toward opposite poles.

Metaphase
Microtubule spindle apparatus attaches to chromosomes. Chromosomes align along spindle equator.

Anaphase
Sister chromatids separate and move to opposite poles.

Telophase
Chromatids arrive at each pole, and new nuclear membranes form. Cell division begins.

Daughter cells
Cell division complete. Each cell receives chromosomes that are identical to those in original nucleus.

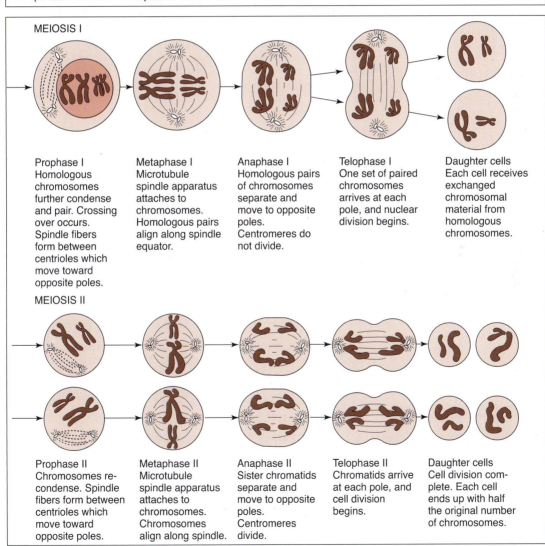

MEIOSIS I

Prophase I
Homologous chromosomes further condense and pair. Crossing over occurs. Spindle fibers form between centrioles which move toward opposite poles.

Metaphase I
Microtubule spindle apparatus attaches to chromosomes. Homologous pairs align along spindle equator.

Anaphase I
Homologous pairs of chromosomes separate and move to opposite poles. Centromeres do not divide.

Telophase I
One set of paired chromosomes arrives at each pole, and nuclear division begins.

Daughter cells
Each cell receives exchanged chromosomal material from homologous chromosomes.

MEIOSIS II

Prophase II
Chromosomes recondense. Spindle fibers form between centrioles which move toward opposite poles.

Metaphase II
Microtubule spindle apparatus attaches to chromosomes. Chromosomes align along spindle.

Anaphase II
Sister chromatids separate and move to opposite poles. Centromeres divide.

Telophase II
Chromatids arrive at each pole, and cell division begins.

Daughter cells
Cell division complete. Each cell ends up with half the original number of chromosomes.

FIGURE 2–14
Mitosis vs. meiosis comparison

Notes:

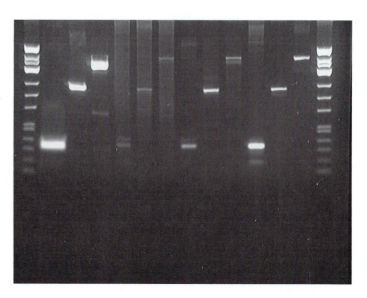

FIGURE 2–15

DNA proofreading (Courtesy of Stratagene, An Agilent Technologies Company. Agilent Technologists, Inc. makes no warranty as to the accuracy of completeness of the foregoing material and hereby disclaims any responsibility therefore.)

KEY CONCEPTS

- A cell is composed of a cell membrane, cytoplasm, organelles, and a nucleus. Each has a distinct function. The cell membrane separates the interior of the cell from the exterior of the cell and surrounding cells. The cytoplasm is the site of chemical reactions within the cell. The organelles aid in the functioning of the cell. The nucleus is the brain of metabolic activity and cell division.

- There are four types of organic compounds: proteins, carbohydrates, lipids, and nucleic acids. Proteins assist in cellular growth and repair; carbohydrates provide energy to the cell; lipids provide energy storage, insulation, and lubrication; and nucleic acids comprise the DNA and RNA of the cell.

- Potassium and sodium are inorganic molecules vital to cell life. These substances serve to maintain osmotic pressure within the cell.

- Mitosis is the process of cell division in which the nucleus and the cytoplasm divide to form two identical cells.

- Meiosis is the process of cell division for the purpose of reproduction.

- Cells utilize enzymes to proofread their work and correct mistakes that may occur during the DNA replication process.

American Society of Radiologic Technologists

CURRICULUM

The material presented in this chapter reflects the following area(s) of the ASRT Curriculum Guide:

Topic:

Radiation Biology

Content:

   I. Introduction

REVIEW QUESTIONS & EXERCISES

Crossword Puzzle

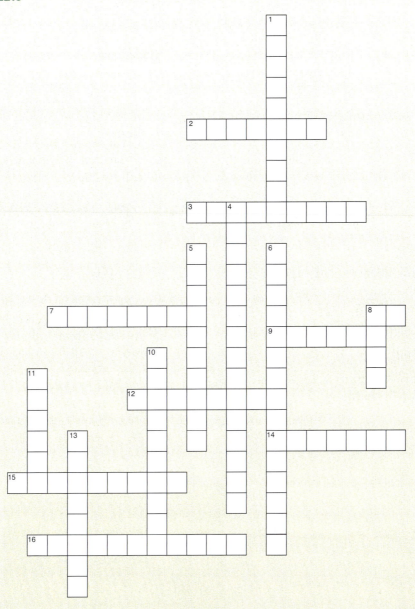

Across

2. Possessing two sets of chromosomes.

3. The halves into which the chromosome is longitudinally divided, which are held together by the centromere and move to opposite poles of a dividing cell during anaphase.

7. The first stage of mitosis or meiosis when chromosomes become visible.

8. The gap or growth period following the replication of DNA and prior to mitosis.

9. A complex organic protein that accelerates chemical reactions.

12. Any living entity.

14. Cell division of germ cells, which consists of two cell divisions but only one replication of DNA.

15. The stage of mitosis where chromosomes are arranged.

16. RNA that binds amino acids to ribosomes during protein synthesis.

Down

1. The destructive phase of metabolism, in which complex substances are changed into simpler substances.

4. Nucleic acid that controls protein synthesis.

5. The period between cell division, known as the resting stage, when DNA is being synthesized.

6. A two-layered membrane that surrounds the cell nucleus.

8. The basic unit of heredity that has a specific location on chromosome.

10. The linear thread of a cell nucleus.

11. Period of synthesis or replication.

13. A stage in mitosis and meiosis between metaphase and telophase in which chromatids migrate toward opposite poles of the cell.

Matching

Match the definition in the right column with the correct term from the left column.

_____ 1. Anabolism

_____ 2. Autosome

_____ 3. Centromere

_____ 4. Chromatin

_____ 5. Deoxyribonucleic acid (DNA)

_____ 6. Duplication

_____ 7. G_1

_____ 8. Gamete

_____ 9. Haploid

_____ 10. Macromolecule

_____ 11. Messenger RNA

_____ 12. Mitosis

_____ 13. Nucleolus

_____ 14. Polymer

_____ 15. Protoplasm

_____ 16. Ribosomal RNA

_____ 17. Telophase

a. RNA that carries amino acids to ribosomes for assisting in protein synthesis

b. Having half the diploid number of chromosomes found in somatic cells

c. Any chromosome that is other than the sex chromosome

d. The gap or growth period following the replication of DNA and prior to mitosis

e. A molecule created by combining two or more of the same molecules

f. The construction phase of metabolism, when a cell takes the substances from blood that are necessary for repair and growth and converts them into cytoplasm

g. The constricted area of the chromosome that separates the chromosome into two arms

h. Spherical body in the cell nucleus that holds nuclear RNA

i. The final stage of mitosis or meiosis, during which there is reconstruction of the nuclear membrane and cell cytoplasm divides, giving birth to two daughter cells

j. Type of cell division involving somatic cells in which a parent cell divides to create two daughter cells that contain the same chromosome number and DNA content as the parent

k. A material in the nucleus that contains genetic information

l. A polymer composed of deoxyribo-nucleotides arranged in a double helix

m. A chromosome mutation in which either one or both segments of a chromosome join to another chromosome

n. The mature male or female reproductive cell

o. A large molecule

p. A colloidal structure of organic and inorganic materials and water that form the living cell

q. RNA that exists in ribosomes and assists in protein synthesis

Multiple Choice

1. Two or more tissues combined to perform a specific function is a definition for:
   - a. cells.
   - b. tissues.
   - c. organs.
   - d. systems.

2. _____ assist in growth, construct new tissues, and repair injured or worn-out cells.
   - a. Proteins
   - b. Enzymes
   - c. Lipids
   - d. Carbohydrates

3. The location of genetic information is in the:
   - a. cell membrane.
   - b. endoplasmic reticulum.
   - c. mitochondria.
   - d. nucleus.

4. Which of the following is the RNA nucleotide base that pairs with adenine in DNA synthesis?
   - a. thymine
   - b. uracil
   - c. guanine
   - d. cytosine

5. The normal diploid or 2n number in humans is:
   - a. 11
   - b. 23
   - c. 46
   - d. 46 pair

6. In which phase of mitosis do the chromosomes line up at the equator of the cell?
   - a. prophase
   - b. metaphase
   - c. anaphase
   - d. telophase

7. During meiosis, or reduction division:
   - a. the cell divides twice in succession, but chromosomes are duplicated only one time.
   - b. the cell divides twice in succession, and chromosomes are duplicated twice.
   - c. the cell divides only once, and chromosomes are duplicated only one time.
   - d. the cell divides only once, but chromosomes are duplicated twice.

EXPLORING THE WEB

1. Search the Web by using the key terms mitosis and meiosis. Can you find any demonstrations of these concepts?

   _____

   _____

   _____

   _____

2. Search the Web for organic compounds. Describe the roles and functions of these compounds in the human body.

   _____

   _____

   _____

   _____

3. Search the Web for inorganic compounds. Describe the roles and functions of these substances in the human body.

_____

_____

_____

_____

CASE STUDY

You have been asked to speak to a group of radiography students about mitosis and meiosis. Compare and contrast the two, discussing the stages involved. Provide a brief summary.

_____

_____

_____

_____

_____

_____

CHAPTER 3

Cellular Effects of Radiation

KEY TERMS

Bystander effects

Deletion

Dicentric

Division delay

Dose-response relationship (curve)

Free radical

HeLa

Interphase death

Linear dose-response curve

Linear quadratic dose-response curve

Linear energy transfer (LET)

Mutation

Nonthreshold

Oxygen effect

Point mutation

Radiolysis

Radiosensitivity

OBJECTIVES

Upon completion of this chapter, the reader should be able to:

- Examine the physical and biologic factors affecting cell radiosensitivity
- Inspect the direct and indirect effects of radiation
- Evaluate the radiolysis of water
- Explain the irradiation of macromolecules
- Analyze the types of dose-response relationships
- Discuss the target theory
- Explain cell survival curves

Notes:

RADIOSENSITIVITY OF CELLS

When radiation damage appears at the whole body level, this is a result of damage to organ **systems**, which are a consequence of radiation damage to cells of that particular system.

Tissue system cells are distinguished by their rate of cell division (proliferation), and their stage of development. *Immature cells are also known as undifferentiated, precursor, or stem cells.* As stated previously in the Law of Bergonie and Tribondeau, immature cells are significantly more radiosensitive than are mature cells.

Cells that are considered highly radiosensitive include: lymphocytes, spermatogonia, erythroblasts, and intestinal crypt cells.

Cells that have an intermediate radiosensitivity include: endothelial cells, osteoblasts, spermatids, and fibroblasts.

Cells that have low radiosensitivity include: muscle and nerve cells, and chondrocytes.

Cell radiosensitivity depends upon what part of the cell cycle the cell is in. Mitosis, and the passage from late G_1 into early S-phase, are judged the most radiosensitive phases of the cell cycle. Mid- to late S-phase is considered to be the most radioresistant cell cycle phase. (See Figure 3–1.)

Numerous experiments have determined that the nucleus of a cell is considerably more radiosensitive than is the cytoplasm of the cell. DNA is the most radiosensitive part of the cell. RNA radiosensitivity is intermediate between that of DNA and protein. Chromosome-produced radiation damage can be analyzed during the metaphase portion of the cell cycle.

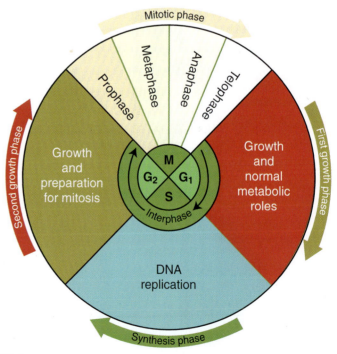

FIGURE 3–1
Cell cycle

Physical and Biologic Factors

When a cell is irradiated, three events may occur. These include the slowing down of cell mitosis, **interphase death**, and cell death.

It has been proven in experiments that low doses of radiation delay cell mitosis in humans. The specific cause for this slow-down, known as **division delay**, is unknown.

Interphase death, which is cell death before entering mitosis, depends on which cell is irradiated. Highly mitotic cells demonstrate interphase death at doses lower than cells that are not highly mitotic. It is theorized that when there is a change in the cell membrane, electrolytes become imbalanced. The consequence for cells that do not divide repetitively, or that divide numerous times resulting in dead cells being produced, is failure of cell reproduction.

When noting biologic changes that occur in cells caused by irradiating them, the following should be emphasized:

- Radiation interaction with cells has to do with chance and probability. The radiation may or may not interact; if it does interact, there may or may not be cell damage.
- The first deposit of radiation is given very rapidly, approximately within 10^{-17} seconds.
- The interaction of radiation within the cell is random.
- It cannot be determined if visible changes to cells, tissues, and organs are caused by radiation or other sources.
- Radiation doses to cells cause biologic changes only following a period of time that is dose dependent, and may vary from minutes to years.

The factors affecting cell response include linear energy transfer (LET), relative biologic effectiveness (RBE), and oxygen enhancement ratio (OER).

Linear Energy Transfer   **Linear energy transfer (LET)** describes a measure of the rate at which energy is deposited as a charged particle travels through matter. LET is described in terms of keV/micrometer. LET is a function of the physical characteristics of radiation, that is, mass and charge. As electromagnetic radiation (x- and gamma-rays) produce few and sparse interactions because of their fast-moving electrons (which have negligible mass and a –1 charge), they are regarded as low LET radiation. These lose or deposit their energy at a much lower rate when passing through tissue.

Compared with electromagnetic radiation, particulate radiations (for example, alpha particles and neutrons), which are highly ionizing and have substantial mass and/or charge, are more likely to interact with tissue. These radiations lose their energy quickly, and produce numerous ionizations within a very short distance. Alpha and neutron radiation are thus considered high LET radiations.

The higher the LET of radiation, the greater the chance for a biologic interaction. Diagnostic X-rays, which have an LET of approximately 3 keV/mm, are considered to be low when compared with all radiations.

TABLE 3–1

Types of Radiation with Corresponding LET Values

Radiation Type	LET (keV/µm)
Cobalt-60	0.25
1 MeV electrons	0.3
Diagnostic X-rays	3.0
10 MeV protons	4.0
2.5 MeV neutrons	20.0
5 MeV alpha particle	100.0
Heavy nuclei	1000.0

Table 3–1 lists average LET values for different types of radiation.

Relative Biologic Effectiveness   The relative effect of LET is quantitatively described by the **relative biologic effectiveness (RBE).** RBE is a comparison of a dose of test radiation to a dose of 250 keV X-ray that produces the same biologic response. RBE is expressed as follows:

$$RBE = \frac{\text{dose in rads from 250 keV X-ray necessary to produce a given effect}}{\text{dose in rads of test radiation necessary to produce the same effect}}$$

The constant is the biologic response, not the radiation dose. The RBE measures the biologic effectiveness of radiations having different LETs.

EXAMPLE

When rats are irradiated with 250 kEv X-rays, 300 rad are required to cause death. If these rats are irradiated with heavy nuclei, only 100 rad are necessary. Calculate the RBE for the heavy nuclei.

$$RBE = \frac{300 \text{ rad}}{100 \text{ rad}} = 3$$

Factors that influence RBE include radiation type, cell or tissue type, physiologic condition, biologic result being examined, and the radiation dose rate.

In comparing LET and RBE, as LET increases, RBE increases also. (See Figure 3–2.) Accordingly, low LET radiations have a low RBE, and high LET radiations have a high RBE. Diagnostic X-rays are considered to have an RBE of approximately 1.

Oxygen Enhancement Ratio   The response of biologic tissue to radiation is greater when irradiated in the oxygenated, or aerobic,

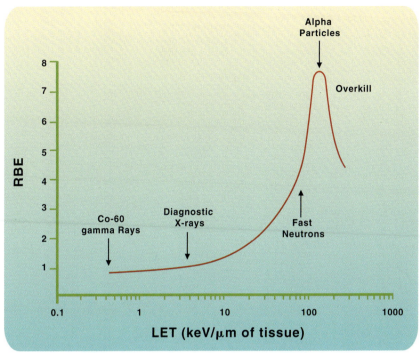

FIGURE 3–2
RBE vs. LET

state than when irradiated in anoxic or hypoxic conditions. This is known as the **oxygen effect**. The oxygen effect is described numerically by the oxygen enhancement ratio (OER). OER is defined as the dose of radiation that produces a given biologic response under anoxic conditions divided by the dose of radiation that produces the same biologic response under aerobic conditions. It is theorized that oxygen is needed in order for free radicals to form during ionization of water. Without the free radicals, hydrogen peroxide is not formed, and thus cell damage is reduced.

$$OER = \frac{\text{dose that produces a given biologic response under anoxic conditions}}{\text{dose that produces the same biologic response under aerobic conditions}}$$

OER depends on LET. The OER is most pronounced for low LET radiation, and is less effective with high LET radiation. For mammal cells, OER is between 2 and 3. The OER for high LET radiations is between 1.2 and 1.7.

Because of the physical differences between high and low LET radiation, the quantity of damage done by high LET radiation would be beyond repair. Thus, having oxygen present would not intensify the response to radiation to the same magnitude, as would be the case with low LET radiation (Figure 3–3).

EXAMPLE

Rat tumors are irradiated using hypoxic conditions. The tumor control dose is 5,000 rad. Irradiating the tumors under aerobic conditions requires a control dose of 1,000 rad. What is the OER for this system?

$$OER = \frac{5,000}{1,000} = 5$$

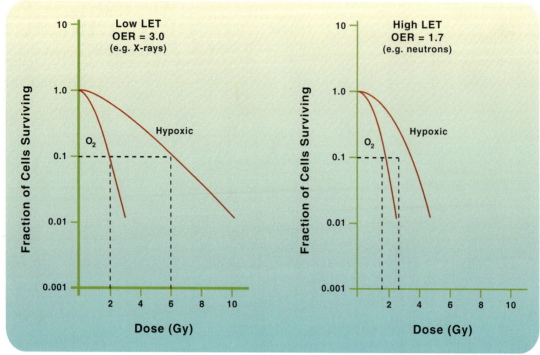

FIGURE 3–3
Oxygen effect on LET

Notes: _____

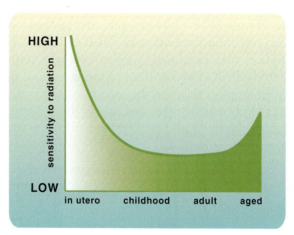

FIGURE 3–4
Age and radiosensitivity

Age   Age influences radiosensitivity. We are most radiosensitive before birth. Radiosensitivity declines until maturity, the time when we are most radioresistant. With old age, humans again tend to become more radiosensitive (Figure 3–4). These concepts are consistent with the Law of Bergonie and Tribondeau.

Direct and Indirect Effects of Radiation

When radiation interactions occur in a cell, these ionizations and excitations develop either in macromolecules (such as DNA) or in their suspension medium (such as water). Depending on the location of the interaction, it is termed either direct or indirect.

Direct interaction is said to take place when an original ionizing incident happens on that macromolecule (for example, DNA, RNA, protein, or enzyme). If a macromolecule becomes ionized, it is considered abnormal and thus damaged.

Indirect interaction occurs if the initial ionizing incident takes place on a distant noncritical molecule, which then transfers the ionization of energy to another molecule.

INTERACTIONS WITH RADIATION

Although it is impossible to determine whether ionizations of molecules occur through direct versus indirect effects, as the human body is approximately 75% water, it is theorized that most radiation actions with humans are indirect. The response to cell irradiation is also determined by the dose in rads.

Radiolysis of Water

With the human body being approximately 75% water, it follows that the irradiation of water is involved in the majority of interactions involving radiation. Although DNA is the most critical target of radiation, it is the irradiation of water, which causes indirect effects, that is the principal cause of effects from radiation. If water is irradiated, the water is ionized, and separates into other molecular products. This is called the **radiolysis** of water.

When an atom of water is irradiated, this ionizes the water, and produces a free radical (Figure 3–5). A **free radical** is an uncharged molecule that contains a single unpaired electron in its outermost or valence shell, which makes it chemically unstable and highly reactive.

Even though free radicals have an estimated life of less than 1 millisecond, they are able to diffuse through the cell and interact at a distant site. They have excess energy that can be moved to other

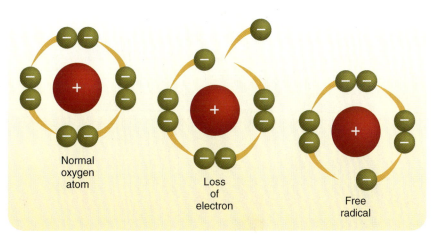

Normal
oxygen
atom

Loss
of
electron

Free
radical

FIGURE 3–5
Formation of free radical of oxygen

Notes:

molecules and interfere with bonds at sites distant from the original ionizing incident.

Reactions of water include:

$$H_2O + radiation = HOH^+ + e^-$$
$$H_2O + e^- = HOH^-$$
$$HOH^+ = H^+ + OH^*$$
$$HOH^- = OH^- + H^*$$
$$OH^* + OH^* = H_2O_2$$

The result of the radiolysis of water is the development of an ion pair, H^+ and OH^-, and two free radicals, H^* and OH^*. The ions can recombine and form a normal water molecule, or they can react chemically and damage cell macromolecules.

The OH^*, which is the hydroxyl free radical, along with hydrogen peroxide (H_2O_2) are estimated to cause approximately two-thirds of all radiation damage following the radiolysis of water.

Ionization occurs when an atom has an extra electron, or has had an electron removed. If an ion has more electrons than it does protons, it is designated with a negative sign. If an ion has more protons than electrons, it is designated with a positive sign.

Irradiation of Macromolecules

The occurrence of molecular derangements or lesions may be classified as either effects on macromolecules or effects on water. Irradiating macromolecules gives very different results when compared to the irradiating of water (Figure 3–6). If macromolecules are exposed to

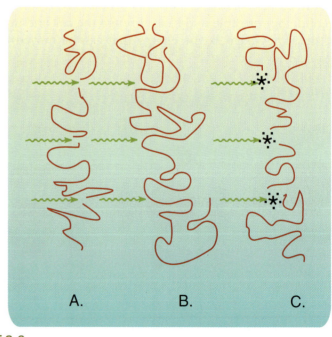

A.   B.   C.

FIGURE 3–6
Macromolecule mutations

ionizing radiation *in vitro* (outside the body or cell), a significant dose of radiation is needed to produce a measurable effect. Irradiating macromolecules *in vivo* (inside the living cell) shows that when cells are in their natural conditions, they are much more radiosensitive.

The three primary effects of irradiating macromolecules *in vitro* include main-chain scission, cross-linking, and point lesions.

Main-Chain Scission   Main-chain scission occurs when the thread or backbone of the long-chain molecule is broken (Figure 3–6A). This results in the long-chain molecule being reduced to numerous smaller molecules, which can still be macromolecular in nature. Not only is the size of the macromolecule reduced, but its viscosity (thickness) is also reduced.

Cross-linking   Certain macromolecules have spur-like extensions off the main chain. Others develop these spurs after being irradiated. After being irradiated, these spurs can act as if they had sticky material on their ends. This stickiness causes the macromolecule to connect to another macromolecule, or to another section of the same molecule. This is termed cross-linking. Viscosity is increased by radiation-produced molecular cross-linking (Figure 3–6B).

Point Lesions   Irradiating macromolecules may result in disturbance of single chemical bonds, which create molecular lesions or point lesions. Point lesions may cause slight molecular changes, which in turn cause the cell to function incorrectly (Figure 3–6C). At low doses of radiation, point lesions are regarded to be the cellular radiation damage that is responsible for the late radiation effects, which are observed at the whole-body level.

Irradiating macromolecules may result in either death of the cell or late effects. Throughout the cell cycle, proteins are constantly being created and occur in greater numbers than the nucleic acids. Abundant copies of unique protein molecules always exist in the cell. These factors allow proteins to be more radioresistant than the nucleic acids. Also, numerous copies of m-RNA and t-RNA exist in the cell, although they are not as plentiful as the protein molecules. Conversely, DNA molecules, having their distinctive base arrangements, are not so numerous. Because of this, DNA is considered the most radiosensitive macromolecule. RNA **radiosensitivity** is midway between that of DNA and protein macromolecules.

There can be visible chromosome abnormalities or cytogenetic damage if the radiation damage to the DNA is intense enough. DNA can be injured without producing visible chromosomal aberrations. Even though this damage is reversible, it can lead to death of the cell and ultimately destroy tissues or organs.

Metabolic activity can also be affected by DNA damage. The primary characteristic of radiation-induced malignancies is the uncontrolled reproduction of cells. If germ cells receive DNA damage, the response may be detected in future offspring (Figure 3–7). In Figure 3–7, A–D illustrate DNA aberrations that are all reversible types of damage. They may involve the sequence of bases being

Notes:

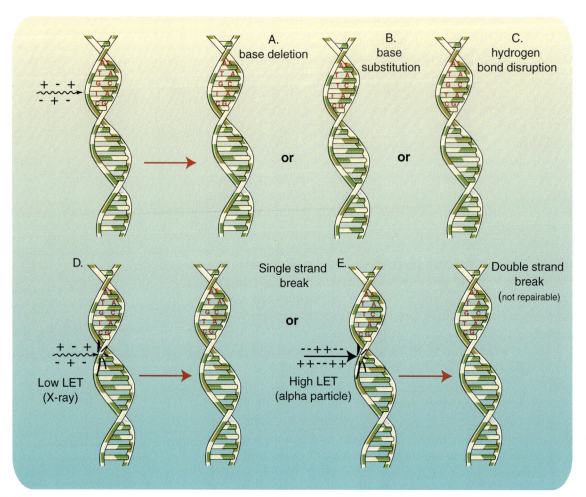

FIGURE 3–7
DNA aberrations

changed, thus changing the triplet code of codons. This is considered a genetic mutation at the molecular level.

The damage type shown in Figure 3–7E also involves the change of or loss of a base. This type of damage also destroys the triplet code, and may not be reversible; this is considered a genetic mutation.

These molecular genetic **mutations** are termed **point mutations**, and are common with low LET radiations. Point mutations may be either of minor or major significance to the cell. A very major effect of these point mutations would be the genetic code being incorrectly transferred to daughter cells.

Single-Hit Chromosome Aberrations

When chromosomes are irradiated, the interaction can be either direct or indirect. The result of either interaction is called a hit. Chromosome hits cause a visible chromosome change (Figure 3–8). Such a hit would mean that numerous molecular bonds had been interfered with, and that several chains of DNA had been severed. Chromosome hits represent critical DNA damage.

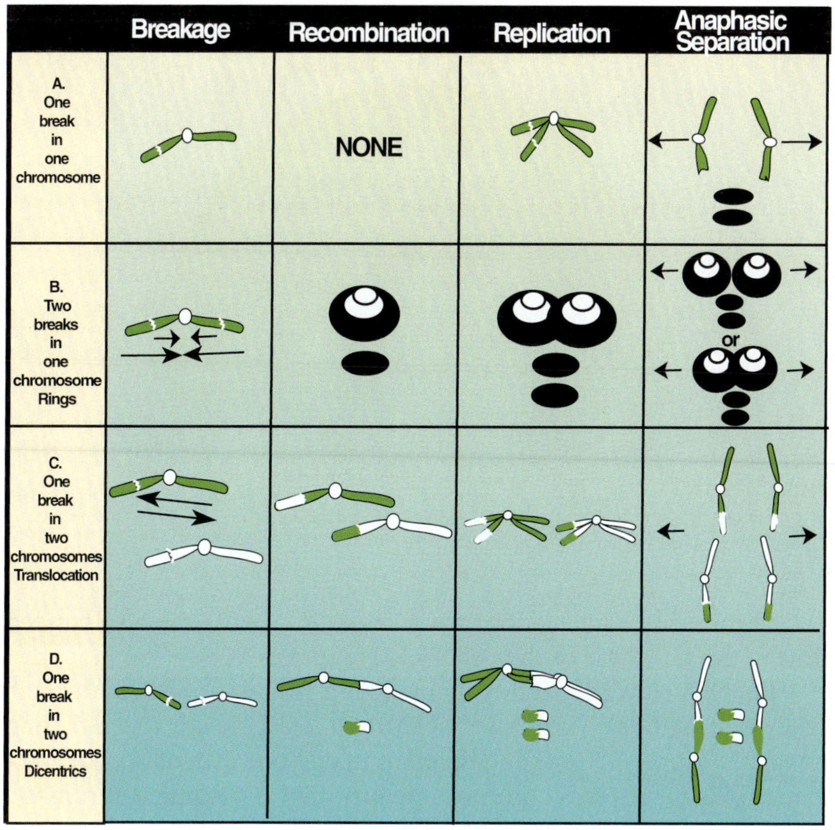

Notes:

	Breakage	Recombination	Replication	Anaphasic Separation
A. One break in one chromosome		NONE		
B. Two breaks in one chromosome Rings				or
C. One break in two chromosomes Translocation				
D. One break in two chromosomes Dicentrics				

FIGURE 3–8

Chromosome aberrations (Reproduced with permission from Bushberg, J. T., Seibert, J. A., Leidholt, E. M., & Boone, J. M. [2001]. *The essential physics of medical imaging* [2nd ed.]. Philadelphia: Lippincott, Williams and Wilkins.)

This figure demonstrates the single-hit effects caused by radiation during the G_1 portion of the cell cycle (Figure 3–9).

If there is breakage of a chromatid, this is termed chromatid **deletion**. During the S-phase of the cell cycle, the deletion and the remaining chromosome are replicated. The chromosome abnormality that is seen during metaphase is a normal-appearing chromosome with material missing from the ends of two sister chromatids and two acentric fragments. Such fragments are called isochromatids.

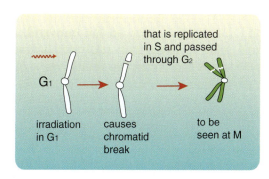

FIGURE 3–9

Single hit effect G_1 (Reprinted with permission from Bushong. [1997]. *Radiologic science for technologists* [6th ed.]. St. Louis: Mosby.)

Notes:

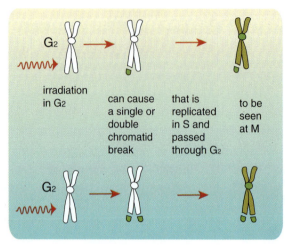

FIGURE 3–10

Single hit effects G$_2$ (Reprinted with permission from Bushong. [1997]. *Radiologic science for technologists* [6th ed.]. St. Louis: Mosby.)

Chromosome aberrations from single-hit events can also happen during the G$_2$ phase of the cell cycle (Figure 3–10).

There is a low probability that ionizing radiation will pass through sister chromatids to produce isochromatids. Instead, the radiation normally causes a chromatid deletion in just one arm of the chromosome. This results in a chromosome arm that is missing a chromatid fragment and consequently is missing genetic material.

Multi-Hit Chromosome Aberrations

It is theorized that human chromosomes have more than a single target. Thus, it is feasible for a single chromosome to receive more than one hit (Figure 3–11). These multi-hit aberrations are not unusual.

During the G$_1$ phase of the cell cycle, if two hits occur on one chromosome, **ring** chromosomes are produced. When neighboring

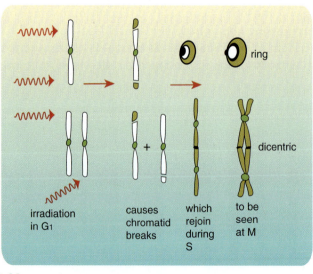

FIGURE 3–11

Multi-hit chromosome aberrations (Reprinted with permission from Bushong. [1997]. *Radiologic science for technologists* [6th ed.]. St. Louis: Mosby.)

Notes:

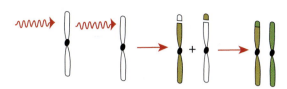

FIGURE 3-12
Reciprocal translocations (Reprinted with permission from Bushong. [1997]. *Radiologic science for technologists* [6th ed.]. St. Louis: Mosby.)

chromosomes each suffer one hit and then recombine, this produces **dicentric** (a chromosome with two centers or two centromeres) fragments. The quality of the stickiness present at the severed chromosome is the determining factor for the joining of the chromatid. (See Figure 3–11.)

During the G_2 phase of the cell cycle, similar chromosomal abnormalities can occur. These types of aberrations are rare, as they require that the same chromosome is hit two or more times, or that neighboring chromosomes are hit and join together.

Multi-hit chromosomal aberrations are representative of major cell damage. During mitosis, either the acentric fragments will be lost, or they will be attracted to just one of the two daughter cells, as they are not connected to a spindle fiber. This results in one or both daughter cells missing significant genetic information.

Reciprocal Translocations

Reciprocal **translocations** are multi-hit chromosomal aberrations. If chromosomes experience this type of alteration, they do not lose any genetic material, but instead the genes become rearranged. This results in all genetic codes being available, but sequenced incorrectly (Figure 3–12).

At the doses received in diagnostic radiology, only single-hit types of chromosomal aberrations are seen. If the radiation dose is not known, the approximate chromosomal aberration frequency will be: two single-hit aberrations/rad/1,000 cells, and one multi-hit aberration/ 10 rad/1,000 cells.

DOSE-RESPONSE RELATIONSHIPS

Dose-response relationships, also referred to as dose-response curves, are a graphical relationship between observed effects (response) from radiation and dose of radiation received (Figure 3–13).

Dose-response curves differ in two ways:

1. They are either linear or nonlinear.
2. They are either threshold or nonthreshold.

Linear means that an observed response is directly proportional to the dose.

EXAMPLE

Doubling the dose of radiation would double the response.

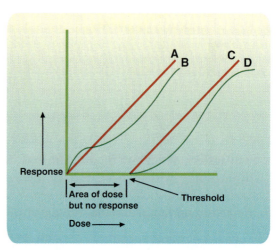

FIGURE 3–13
Dose-response relationships

Nonlinear means that an observed response is not directly proportional to the dose.

EXAMPLE

Doubling the dose of radiation does not double the response.

Threshold assumes that there is a radiation level reached below which there would be no effects observed. **Nonthreshold** assumes that any radiation dose produces an effect.

Diagnostic radiology is primarily concerned with linear, nonthreshold dose-response relationships.

Linear-Dose-Response Relationships

Because dose-response relationships A and B intercept the dose (x) axis at either zero or on the y-axis, they are considered linear, nonthreshold.

All **linear dose-response relationships** exhibit an effect regardless of the dose. This is demonstrated by relationship A. Even at zero dose, A exhibits a measurable response, R_A. This R_A is termed the ambient or natural response. Dose-response relationships C and D intercept the dose (x) axis at a dose value greater than zero. Thus, C and D are considered linear, threshold. At doses below the respective C and D values, no response would be anticipated.

Leukemia, breast cancer, and other genetic damage are believed to follow the linear dose-response relationship.

Linear Quadratic Dose-Response Curves

In 1980, the Committee on the Biological Effects of Ionizing Radiation (BEIR Committee) concluded that the effects of low doses of low LET radiation follow a **linear quadratic dose-response**

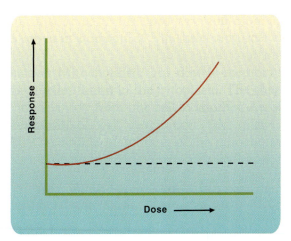

FIGURE 3–14
Linear quadratic dose-response curve

relationship (Figure 3–14). At low doses, the curve is linear. At higher doses, the curve becomes curvilinear. The curve is nonthreshold.

The portion of the curve where increases in dose show no or little increase in effect is named the toe. The shoulder is considered the area of the curve in which a leveling off occurs, again demonstrating no or little increase in effect.

This model underestimates the low dose effect of radiation, as the linear part of the curve is somewhat leveled off or flattened.

In 1990, with 10 additional years of human data, the BEIR committee revised its radiation risk estimates and adopted the linear, nonthreshold dose-response relationship as most relevant.

Current radiation protection guidelines are established using the linear nonthreshold dose-response relationship model.

Nonlinear Dose-Response Relationships The sigmoid dose-response curve is applied predominately to the high dose effects observed in radiotherapy (Figure 3–15). **Sigmoid** means s-shaped. There is normally a threshold below which no observable effects occur.

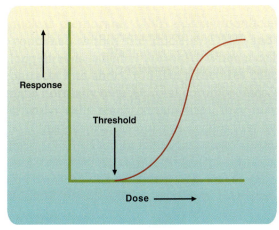

FIGURE 3–15
Sigmoid dose-response curve

Notes:

With a sigmoid dose-response curve, there is a nonlinear relationship between dose and effect, meaning that the effect is not directly proportional to the dose.

TARGET THEORY

As cells contain a profusion of molecules, radiation damage to these molecules is not likely to result in significant cell injury because additional molecules are present to assist in cell survival. However, there are molecules that are not in abundance which are considered necessary for cell survival. Irradiating these could have serious consequences, because there may not be others available to maintain cell survival.

This idea of a sensitive critical molecule is the foundation for the target theory. According to the target theory, there will be cell death only if the cell's target molecule is inactivated. It is theorized that DNA is the critical molecular target.

The target is regarded to be the area of the cell that contains the target molecule. Because radiation interaction with cells is random, target interactions also occur randomly. The radiation shows no favoritism toward the target molecule.

When a target is irradiated, this is considered a hit. Both direct and indirect effects cause hits (Figure 3–16). Direct versus indirect hits are not distinguishable.

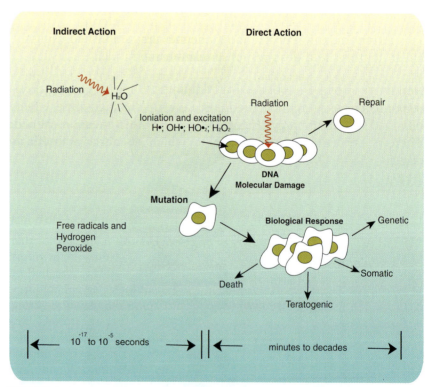

FIGURE 3–16

Target theory (Reproduced with permission from Bushberg, J. T., Seibert, J. A., Leidholt, E. M., & Boone, J. M. [2001]. *The essential physics of medical imaging* [2nd ed.]. Philadelphia: Lippincott, Williams and Wilkins.)

With low LET radiation in an anoxic condition, chances for a hit on the target molecule are low because of the large distances between ionizing events.

In an aerobic state with low LET radiation, the indirect effect is intensified, as more free radicals are formed, and the volume of action surrounding each interaction is enlarged. This increases the likelihood of a hit.

Using high LET radiation, ionization distances are so close together that there is a high probability that a direct hit will take place, probably even higher than for the low LET, indirect effect.

Adding oxygen to high LET radiation will probably not result in additional hits, as the high LET has already produced the maximum number of hits possible.

Bystander Effect

Treatment of cells with low doses of radiation results in the release of specific factors outside the cell that seem to be responsible for biological changes in cells not directly exposed to radiation. These are called **bystander effects**. It has also been shown that subjecting cells to stresses, such as oxidative damage and radiation, induces the selective release of cell surface proteins by a process of regulated "shedding," or proteolysis.

Proteolysis is responsible for the generation of numerous biologically active molecules such as growth factors and cytokines.

According to the target theory of radiation-induced effects, a central tenet of radiation biology, DNA damage occurs during or very shortly after irradiation of the nuclei in targeted cells, and the potential for biological consequences can be expressed within one or two cell generations. A range of evidence has now emerged that challenges the classical effects resulting from targeted damage to DNA. These effects have also been termed "nontargeted" and include radiation-induced bystander effects, genomic instability, adaptive response, low-dose hyper-radiosensitivity (HRS), delayed reproductive death, and induction of genes by radiation. An essential feature of "nontargeted" effects is that they do not require a direct nuclear exposure by irradiation to be expressed, and they are particularly significant at low doses. This evidence suggests a new paradigm for radiation biology that challenges the universality of target theory. The radiation-induced bystander effect is the phenomenon whereby cellular effects such as sister chromatid exchanges, chromosome aberrations, apoptosis, micronucleation, transformation, mutations, differentiation and changes of gene expression are expressed in unirradiated neighboring cells near to an irradiated cell or cells. The bystander effect cannot be comprehensively explained on the basis of a single cell reaction. It is well known that an organism is composed of different cell types that interact as functional units in a way to maintain normal tissue function. Radiation effects at the tissue level under normal conditions prove that individual cells cannot be considered as an isolated functional unit within most tissues

Notes:

of a multicellular organism. Experimental models, which maintain tissue-like intercellular cell signaling and 3-D structure, are essential for proper understanding of the bystander effect. Only a few papers have been published on bystander effects in multicellular system.

With the exception of abscopal effects and clastogenic factors in the blood plasma of patients undergoing radiation therapy, little evidence of a bystander effect under *in vivo* conditions is available. The only experimental work which deals with the bystander effect under *in vivo* conditions is from Watson and coauthors, who utilized a bone marrow transplantation protocol to demonstrate that genomic instability could be induced in bystander cells; a mixture of irradiated and non-irradiated cells, distinguished by a cytogenetic marker, was transplanted into CBA/H mice, and genomic instability was demonstrated in the progeny of the non-irradiated cells.

CELL SURVIVAL CURVES

Cellular sensitivity studies began in the middle 1950s with Puck and Marcus. They performed *in vitro* studies using **HeLa** cells. Their initial study was on failure of reproduction in which they exposed HeLa cells to differing radiation doses and then totaled the number of colonies formed.

This information may be illustrated graphically by plotting the radiation doses on a linear scale on the x-axis, and plotting the fraction of surviving cells on a logarithmic scale on the y-axis. This graphical representation of the relationship between dose and surviving cells is a cell survival curve.

It was stated previously that radiation interaction is random in nature. Therefore, we must determine how many hits are necessary to cause cell death. This may be demonstrated by using a cell survival curve.

In simple cells such as bacteria, if there are additional hits to the same cell, these hits do not matter. In complex cells such as human cells, it is theorized that in order to cause cell death, more than one hit is required.

The graphs of simple versus complex cells are very different (Figure 3–17).

Graph A represents a survival curve for simple cells, represented by a straight line. Graph B represents a survival curve for complex cells, represented by a line that displays a shouldered area where effects are not apparent until some targets have received enough multiple hits to be killed. The target theory can be used to explain this shoulder section of the curve.

If there are n number of cell targets, for example, n = 5, all have to be hit for a cell to be killed. Therefore, the cell must receive five sublethal hits to cause cell death; otherwise, the cell will be able to repair itself. The shoulder region of the curve is the area where hits = n − 1 (for example, 5 −1), or four hits for each cell.

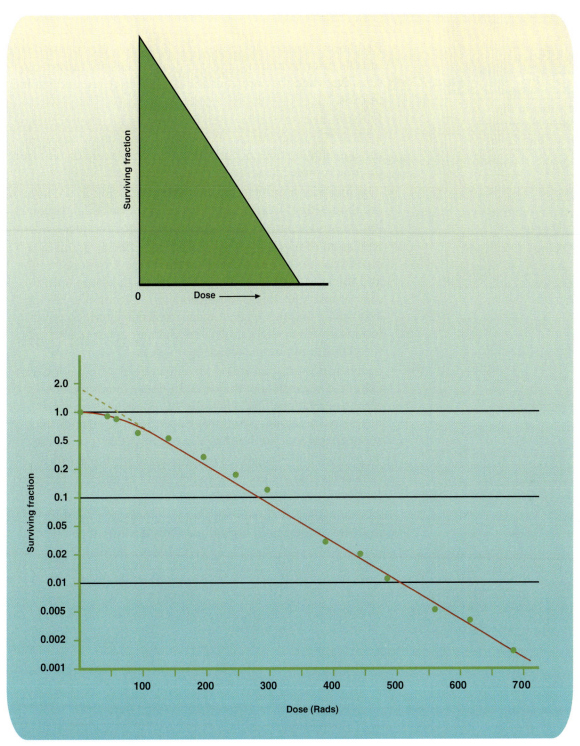

FIGURE 3–17
Simple vs. complex cell survival curves

The shoulder of the cell survival curve shows that some damage must accrue before there can be cell death. The accumulated damage is called sublethal damage. The wider the shoulder, the more sublethal damage the cell can endure.

Notes: _____
_____
_____

Notes: _____

_____

_____

_____

_____

_____

_____

_____

_____

_____

_____

_____

_____

_____

_____

_____

_____

_____

_____

_____

_____

KEY CONCEPTS

- Radiation causes a slowdown in cell mitosis, interphase death of cells prior to mitosis, and cell death. Cells are most radio-sensitive when they are young and when they are undergoing mitosis.

- Direct radiation occurs when the ionizing incident occurs on a particular macromolecule. Indirect radiation occurs when the ionizing incident occurs on a macromolecule distant from the macromolecule affected by the radiation.

- The majority of interactions involving radiation in the human are the result of irradiation of water in the cells that becomes ionized and separates into other molecular products.

- Radiation of macromolecules has three effects: (1) main-chain scission in which the macromolecule is reduced in size and thickness, (2) cross-linking in which the spurs on the macromolecule adhere to other macromolecules, enlarging and thickening the original macromolecule, and (3) point lesions in which slight molecular changes occur that cause the cell to function incorrectly.

- In linear dose-response relationships effects of radiation are exhibited regardless of the dose. In linear quadratic dose-response relationships, a leveling-off effect is observed as doses are increased. Nonlinear dose-response relationships show effects that are not directly proportional to the dose.

- The target theory suggests that there are sensitive critical molecules that are essential to cell survival and that radiation to these cells will result in cell death.

- The cell survival curve identifies the doses that result in inability of the cell to reproduce, thus leading to cell death.

REVIEW QUESTIONS & EXERCISES

Crossword Puzzle

Across

1. Any dose received, regardless of size, which will produce a response.

3. Breakdown of water using radiation.

7. Graph of the relationship between radiation dose and observed response, in which any dose may have a potential effect and there is a direct relationship between radiation dose and observed effect.

9. Letters that represent the first two letters of the patient's first and last names in an experiment conducted by Puck using uterine cervix cells to produce cell cultures.

10. Slow down of cell division due to irradiation.

11. An S-shaped type of dose-response relationship.

Down

2. Graphical representation of relationship between radiation dose and observed response, in which the curve is linear or proportional at low doses, and becomes curvilinear at higher doses.

4. A chromosomal effect that causes a loss of genetic material.

5. The point where a stimulus starts to produce an effect.

6. A comparison of how effective types of radiation are compared with x- and gamma-rays.

8. A mutation that occurs as a result from a change of a single DNA base pair, created by one nucleotide being exchanged for another.

Matching

Match the definition in the right column with the correct term from the left column.

_____ 1. Dicentric

_____ 2. Dose-response relationship (curve)

_____ 3. Free radical

_____ 4. Interphase death

_____ 5. Linear energy transfer (LET)

_____ 6. Mutation

_____ 7. Oxygen effect

_____ 8. Ribosomes

_____ 9. Radiosensitivity

_____ 10. Ring

_____ 11. System

_____ 12. Translocation

a. Altering of a chromosome by a portion of it transferring either to another chromosome or to another section of the same chromosome

b. A chromosome that has two centers or two centromeres

c. A measure of the rate at which energy is deposited from ionizing radiation to soft tissue

d. A structural change or transformation of a chromosome that can be transmitted to offspring

e. A group of cells that perform a particular function

f. A graphical representation of observed effects compared with radiation dose

g. Cell death occurring before mitosis

h. The amount of reaction or response of a cell to radiation

i. Mutation of chromosome causing it to become ring-shaped

j. Enhanced cell response due to aerobic conditions

k. An atom that has an unpaired electron, making it highly reactive

l. Assist in protein synthesis

Multiple Choice

1. Which of the following cell groups are considered highly radiosensitive?
    a. lymphocytes, spermatogonia, erythroblasts, and intestinal crypt cells
    b. endothelial cells, osteoblasts, spermatids, and fibroblasts
    c. muscle and nerve cells, and chondrocytes
    d. muscle cells and osteoblasts

2. Relative biologic effectiveness (RBE):
    a. describes a measure of the rate at which energy is deposited as a charged particle travels through matter.
    b. is a comparison of a dose of test radiation to a dose of 250-keV X-ray that produces the same biologic response.
    c. is defined as the dose of radiation that produces a given biologic response under anoxic conditions divided by the dose of radiation that produces the same biologic response under aerobic conditions.
    d. states that stem cells are more radiosensitive than mature cells.

3. Which of the following body molecules are most commonly acted upon directly by ionizing radiation to produce indirect effects?
    a. lipids   c. carbohydrates
    b. proteins   d. water

4. The types of DNA molecule damage include:
    1. main-chain scission, one side rail broken
    2. main-chain scission, both side rails broken
    3. main-chain scission, resulting in cross-linking
    4. rung breakage, causing bases to separate
    5. a changing or loss of a base

    a. 1 only
    b. 2 and 3 only
    c. 5 only
    d. 1, 2, 3, 4, and 5

5. At low doses of radiation, most cellular radiation damage is the result of:
    a. main-chain scission.   c. point lesions.
    b. cross-linking.   d. gender.

6. Nonthreshold:
    a. means that an observed response is directly proportional to the dose.
    b. means that an observed response is not directly proportional to the dose.
    c. assumes that there is a radiation level reached under which there would be no effects observed.
    d. assumes that any radiation dose produces an effect.

7. According to target theory:
    a. only direct effects can cause hits.
    b. only indirect effects can cause hits.
    c. RNA is considered the critical target.
    d. DNA is considered the critical target.

EXPLORING THE WEB

1. Search the Web for information related to dose-response curves and radiobiology. What additional information can you find?

    _____

    _____

    _____

    _____

2. Search for effects of radiation at the cellular level. Describe the impact radiation has in cells. Discuss the effects of cellular radiation as a treatment for cancer.

    _____

    _____

    _____

    _____

3. Search for radiation therapy. Discuss the concepts of radiation therapy and relate them to the discussion in your text.

    _____

    _____

    _____

    _____

4. Search for more information on the target theory and the oxygen effect.

    _____

    _____

    _____

    _____

CASE STUDY

One of your family members tells you he saw an article on television about radiation dose-response relationships. He asks you to explain this concept for him. Describe dose-response relationships using the terms linear/nonlinear and threshold/nonthreshold.

_____

_____

_____

_____

_____

SECTION 1 REVIEW

MULTIPLE CHOICE

1. The process of cell division of somatic cells is known as:
    - a. mitosis
    - b. synthesis
    - c. meiosis
    - d. reduction division

2. How does oxygen retention affect cell radiosensitivity?
    - a. increases radiosensitivity
    - b. decreases radiosensitivity
    - c. destroys radiosensitivity
    - d. does not affect radiosensitivity

3. What is the name of the molecule that has one or more unpaired electrons and is usually chemically reactive?
    - a. centromere
    - b. polypeptide
    - c. free radical
    - d. ion

4. Which of the following measures the rate of energy lost along the track of an ionizing particle?
    - a. relative biologic effectiveness (RBE)
    - b. linear energy transfer (LET)
    - c. oxygen enhancement ratio (OER)
    - d. cell survival curve

5. Which of the following would be considered most radiosensitive?
    - a. a fetus
    - b. a pediatric patient
    - c. a teenage patient
    - d. an adult patient

6. Of the following stages of mitosis, which is considered the most radiosensitive?
    - a. prophase
    - b. anaphase
    - c. metaphase
    - d. telophase

7. Which of the following describes the shape of a DNA molecule?
    - a. oval
    - b. spherical
    - c. rectangular
    - d. double helix

8. How many matched pairs of chromosomes does a normal human cell contain?
    - a. 11
    - b. 23
    - c. 46
    - d. 47

9. Which stage of cell division is also known as the "resting stage"?
    - a. prophase
    - b. anaphase
    - c. metaphase
    - d. interphase

10. If a DNA base sequence is altered, which of the following would occur?
    - a. a gene mutation
    - b. a gene duplication
    - c. a gene replication
    - d. formation of chromatin

11. Of the following, which are considered the "building blocks" of protein synthesis?
    - a. chromosomes
    - b. genes
    - c. amino acids
    - d. lipids

12. In which area of the cell is the majority of RNA located?
    a. nucleolus
    b. mitochondria
    c. lysosomes
    d. cytoplasm

13. The small areas of the DNA molecule that determine cell characteristics are named:
    a. adenines
    b. pyrimidines
    c. genes
    d. nucleolus

14. Which of the following contains the human hereditary blueprint?
    a. the RNA
    b. the nucleolus
    c. the gene
    d. the ribosome

15. In mitosis, chromosomes split in half. What are these two halves called?
    a. nuclear membranes
    b. chromatids
    c. centromeres
    d. spindle fibers

16. For protein synthesis to occur, messenger RNA (m-RNA) carries information to which of the following?
    a. DNA
    b. t-RNA
    c. chromosome
    d. ribosome

17. Transfer RNA (t-RNA) carries which of the following in order to synthesize protein?
    a. monosaccharides
    b. polysaccharides
    c. genes
    d. amino acids

18. The majority of a cell's genetic information is found where?
    a. nucleus
    b. cytoplasm
    c. t-RNA
    d. nucleolus

19. The process of cell division of reproductive/germ cells is named:
    a. mitosis
    b. meiosis
    c. synthesis
    d. transcription

20. The following is in reference to the single set of chromosomes in a germ cell:
    a. tetrad
    b. haploid number
    c. diploid number
    d. tetroid number

21. Which of the following measures the rate of energy lost along the track of an ionizing particle?
    a. relative biologic effectiveness (RBE)
    b. linear energy transfer (LET)
    c. oxygen enhancement ratio (OER)
    d. cell survival curve

22. What does the term interphase death mean?
    a. Cells die prior to entering interphase.
    b. Cells die prior to leaving interphase.
    c. Cells die in between mitotic phases.
    d. The organism dies.

23. Which of the following terms is used in describing cell damage from radiation that is not sufficient to kill the cell?
    a. sublethal damage
    b. duplication effect
    c. cell division
    d. replication

24. Why is free radical formation considered such a threat to humans?
    a. free radicals produce scatter radiation
    b. free radicals can penetrate any type of shielding
    c. free radicals have been proven to have carcinogenic effects
    d. free radicals have been observed to produce toxic effects

25. According to the target theory, which of the following is thought to be the principal target of cell damage?
    a. RNA
    b. DNA
    c. cytoplasm
    d. ribosomes

26. What does the term "indirect effect" of ionizing radiation refer to?
    a. Genetic effects are produced.
    b. An ionization occurs directly on the target molecule.
    c. An ionization occurs in one location that can produce effects at a distant location.
    d. Organism death occurs.

27. Which of the following is the term used to describe the separation of water into hydrogen and oxygen following irradiation?
    a. duplication
    b. synthesis
    c. radioactivity
    d. radiolysis

28. Which of the following is used for expressing occupational exposure?
    a. rem
    b. rad
    c. roentgen
    d. LET

29. As linear energy transfer (LET) increases, how is relative biologic effectiveness (RBE) affected?
    a. With an increase in LET, RBE also increases.
    b. With an increase in LET, RBE decreases.
    c. With an increase in LET, RBE is neutralized.
    d. RBE is not affected by LET.

30. To correctly make a DNA base pair, guanine must be bonded to:
    a. thymine
    b. cytosine
    c. guanine
    d. adenine

31. The type of irradiation damage most likely to cause abnormalities in base sequences, and thus cell mutation, would be
    a. single-strand breaks
    b. double-strand breaks
    c. cross-linking
    d. base damage

Biological Effects of Radiation Exposure

It is crucial that radiographers study the effects of ionizing radiation. Radiographers must comprehend the potential risks of ionizing radiation by acquiring a thorough understanding of radiation biology. This section discusses the clinical applications of radiation biology.

Effects of radiation exposure that occur within minutes, hours, days, and weeks are termed early effects. In contrast, late effects of radiation exposure occur months and even years later.

The manner in which an organism responds to total body irradiation is determined by the combined response of all the body systems. Because body systems differ in both radiosensitivity and response, total body response is a function of the specific system that is most influenced by the exposure to radiation.

CHAPTER 4

Effects of Initial Exposure to Radiation

KEY TERMS

Aberration

Acentric

Alopecia

Anemia

Anomaly

Atrophy

Crypts of Lieberkuhn

Cytopenia

Dermis

Desquamation

Dicentric

Edema

Epidermis

Erythroblasts

Follicles

Gametes

Granulocytes

Hemopoietic

Inflammation

Karyotype

OBJECTIVES

Upon completion of this chapter, the reader should be able to:

- Discuss the hematologic, gastrointestinal, and central nervous system syndromes
- Describe local tissue damage to the skin, eyes, and gonads
- Explain hematologic and cytogenetic effects

Notes:

ACUTE RADIATION SYNDROMES

After an organism is exposed to acute whole body radiation, it exhibits certain signs, symptoms, and clinical findings. The term **syndrome** is used to show the relationship of the signs and symptoms to a specific type of trauma or disease process. The term total body radiation syndrome is used as the response of an organism to whole body radiation results in specific findings. Even though the syndrome is caused by damage to one specific system, presentation of unique signs and symptoms is caused by damage to more than one body system.

In order for the total body radiation syndrome to be applicable, radiation exposure must happen under the following conditions: 1) an organ must have been exposed acutely, that is, in a matter of seconds or minutes; 2) there must be exposure of the total body area; 3) external penetrating sources, for example, X-rays, gamma-rays, and neutrons, produce the radiation syndromes. Internally deposited radioactive materials do not result in manifestation of the full syndrome.

The main consequence of an acute radiation exposure is shortening of the life span of the organism. This life span shortening is dose dependent. Because the life span of an organism is dramatically decreased after a moderate to high dose of total body radiation (many hundreds or thousands of rads), whole body exposures in this dose range are regarded as instantly fatal.

Organism survival times are expressed as the average survival time. There are variations in survival times between different species and between animals within the same species. Expressing survival time as the average takes these variations into account.

Because of the variations in survival time of a group of animals exposed to the same whole body dose, the relationship of survival of a whole population of the same species exposed to the same dose is expressed as that dose which will kill a certain percentage of the population within a given period of time. For example, the lethal dose required to kill 50% of a population in 30 days is expressed as the **LD50/30**. As humans often survive beyond this 30-day period, the **LD50/60**, or the lethal dose required to kill 50% of a population in 60 days, may be more useful. The LD50/60 is approximately 250–300 rads. The LD50/30 and acute radiation syndromes assume no medical intervention. Table 4–1 lists the LD50/30 doses in rads for various species.

A curve can be made that relates dose to survival time for all mammals exposed to whole body radiation (Figure 4–1). As the dose goes up, the survival time and number of survivors decreases.

In the dose range of 200 R, death occurs in a small percentage of animals, with the survival time being dose dependent. Animals exposed in this range survive a few weeks. Between 1,000 and 10,000 R, average survival time does not appear to be dose dependent. In this range, all animals irradiated survive for about the same time, approximately three to four days, but fewer survive at these doses than at the lower dose. At doses of 10,000 R and above, average survival time becomes dose dependent, with survival rate decreasing to hours or minutes.

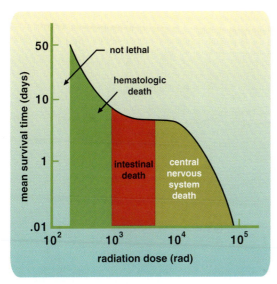

FIGURE 4–1
Mammalian dose survival curve

TABLE 4–1

LD50/30 Values

Species	LD50/30 (rads)
human	250–450
dog	300
monkey	400
chicken	600
frog	700
rabbit	800
rat	900
turtle	1,500
goldfish	2,000
newt	3,000

Notes: _____

In referring to the three regions of the dose response curve, there are three different systems that can result in death to the animal. Other organs and systems have suffered damage, but the principal cause of death is destruction to one specific system. The three defined acute radiation syndromes are named corresponding to failure of that organ system which causes death. These doses are not likely to occur in diagnostic radiology.

In the 100 to 1,000 R range, death is mostly the result of damage to the **hemopoietic** (development of blood cells) system, especially to the bone marrow. Thus, the acute radiation syndrome in this dose range is termed the hematologic, hematopoietic, or bone marrow syndrome.

In the second region of the dose response curve, at approximately 600 to 10,000 R, death is caused by damage to the gastrointestinal system, especially the small intestine. The syndrome within this dose range is known as the gastrointestinal (GI) syndrome.

The third region of the dose response curve, at doses greater than 10,000 R, death is caused by damage to the central nervous system. Thus, this third syndrome is called the central nervous system (CNS) syndrome.

It is important to note two specifics concerning the acute radiation syndrome dose response curve: 1) the dose range figures are obtained from studies of animal response after acute total body exposure, and are not specific for humans. 2) At the higher doses of each range, the syndromes overlap; for example, animals may die from a combination of damage in the bone marrow and GI syndromes. Figure 4–2 shows the interrelationships between the elements of the acute radiation syndrome.

Response Stages

Animal responses to acute total body radiation doses are divided into four stages. The time length of each stage is dose dependent; that is,

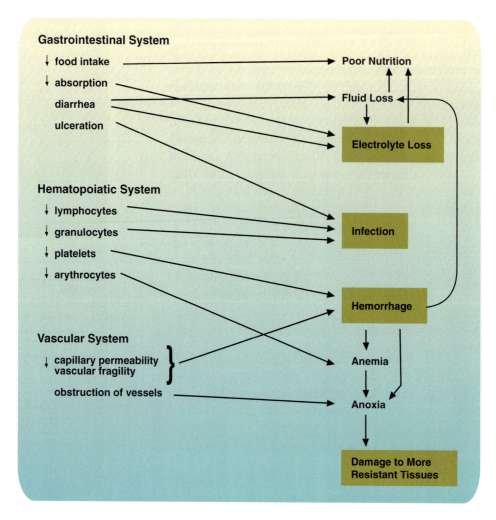

FIGURE 4–2

Acute radiation syndromes (Reproduced with permission from Bushberg, J. T., Seibert, J. A., Leidholt, E. M., & Boone, J. M. [2001]. *The essential physics of medical imaging* [2nd ed.]. Philadelphia: Lippincott, Williams and Wilkins.)

TABLE 4–2

Air Dose Causing Prodromal Symptoms

Dose in Air	Symptoms
1.2 Gy (120 rads)	Anorexia
1.7 Gy (170 rads)	Nausea
2.1 Gy (210 rads)	Vomiting
2.4 Gy (240 rads)	Diarrhea

Pizzarello, D. J., & Witcofski, R. L. (1982). *Medical radiation biology* (2nd ed.). Philadelphia: Lea & Febiger.

the lower the dose, the longer the duration in the stage. Each stage can last from weeks at low doses to minutes at high doses.

The first stage, termed the **prodromal** stage, consists of nausea, vomiting, and diarrhea (also referred to as the N-V-D syndrome). This stage, which can occur with a dose as low as 50 rads, lasts from a few minutes to a few days, being dose dependent (that is, the higher the dose, the shorter the stage). Table 4–2 shows approximate doses in air that will cause various prodromal symptoms in 50% of those people irradiated.

The second stage is known as the **latent** stage. During this period, the animal appears to be symptom-free. In reality, changes are taking place that will either lead to recovery or death. The time length of this stage is also dose dependent, ranging from weeks as in doses below 500 R, to hours or less at doses greater than 10,000 R.

After the latent stage, the animal becomes noticeably ill and shows signs and symptoms of the specific syndrome reflecting the organ system that is damaged. This third stage is called the **manifest** illness stage, and lasts from minutes to weeks depending on the dose.

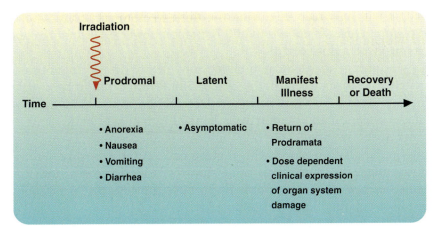

FIGURE 4–3

Acute radiation syndrome phases (From Pizzarello, D. J., & Witcofski, R. L. [1982]. *Medical radiation biology* [2nd ed.]. Philadelphia: Lea & Febiger.)

In the fourth stage, the animal either recovers or dies as a result of the damage sustained from the radiation exposure. Figure 4–3 summarizes the different phases of the acute radiation syndrome.

Even though the timing and manifestation of the signs and symptoms vary among a range of mammals, most mammals show similar signs and symptoms. The survival time after different doses differs greatly among species. In referring back to the LD50/30 values for different species, humans appear to be relatively radiosensitive.

Bone Marrow Syndrome

Bone marrow syndrome, also referred to as the hematologic or hematopoietic syndrome, occurs between 100 and 1,000 R, with death occurring within six to eight weeks in some individuals at a dose of 200 R. No one has survived a dose of 1,000 R. An exposure to this dose would cause death within two weeks. The LD50/60 for humans is estimated to be about 450 R or 250–300 rads, and is in the dose range of this syndrome. Death is caused by destruction of the bone marrow. The mechanism of death is caused by the reduction of red blood cells (RBCs), white blood cells (WBCs), and platelets. Death results from anemia and infection.

The prodromal stage of this syndrome occurs a few hours after exposure and involves nausea and vomiting. The latent stage extends from a few days up to three weeks after exposure, during which time the number of circulating blood cells is not severely depressed. Even though the person looks and feels well, in reality bone marrow stem cells are dying during the prodromal and latent stages. This results in fewer mature cells being produced and lower numbers of cells in the circulating blood. Reduction in blood cell count occurs during the manifest illness stage, which occurs at three to five weeks post-exposure. The signs and symptoms of the manifest illness stage include depression of all blood cell counts (**cytopenia**), which causes **anemia** and infections.

For people suffering with this syndrome, survival time is dose dependent. In the range of 100–300 R, the bone marrow repopulates enough to sustain life in most individuals. A large percentage of these people will fully recover during the third week to six months post-exposure. Doses from 400 to 600 R result in fewer survivors. No one has survived a dose of 1,000 R.

Assuming no medical intervention, death occurs in approximately four to six weeks in the 300 to 500 R range, but in two weeks in the 500 to 1,000 R dose range. Destruction of the bone marrow causes infection and hemorrhage, which ultimately leads to death at these doses. Normally, the bone marrow is filled with cells that supply the circulating blood with mature cells. After exposures in this dose range, the number of bone marrow cells decreases until the bone marrow is no longer able to produce the cells that are needed in the circulating blood to support life.

Gastrointestinal Syndrome

The gastrointestinal (GI) syndrome appears in all animals at doses between 1,000 and 10,000 R. In humans, some symptoms appear at a **threshold dose** of 600 R, with the full syndrome manifest at 1,000 R. Survival time in this syndrome does not vary with dose. Death happens at the same time regardless of dose. Human death occurs within three to ten days without medical support and within approximately two weeks with medical intervention.

Within hours after exposure the prodromal stage occurs. This stage involves nausea and vomiting, cramps, and diarrhea. The latent stage occurs through the fifth day. Following this stage there is a reoccurrence of nausea, vomiting, and diarrhea along with a fever. This is the start of the manifest illness stage, which perseveres from the fifth through the tenth days.

The GI syndrome occurs because of damage to the GI tract and bone marrow. The GI tract lining, especially the small intestine, is damaged by doses in this range. Exposure to radiation causes the **crypts of Lieberkuhn** (the radiosensitive cells that are a precursor to the population of villi cells) to be depleted. This causes the villi to lose cells, and becoming shortened, flattened, and partly or completely denuded.

Because of the villi being flattened, there is decreased absorption of materials across the wall of the intestine. Dehydration occurs from fluids leaking into the GI tract lumen. Systemic infection results from bacteria that pass through the intestinal wall and enter the bloodstream.

During these changes to the GI tract, there is also a depletion of circulating white blood cells because of the bacteria entering the blood stream from the GI tract.

Even though the GI tract attempts regeneration after irradiation, the damage suffered by the bone marrow will likely still cause death. Death results from infection, dehydration, and electrolyte imbalance caused by the damage sustained to the GI tract and bone marrow.

Central Nervous System Syndrome

The central nervous system (CNS) syndrome occurs at doses greater than 5,000 R in humans. Death is usually within hours, but may occur two to three days post-exposure. Depending on the dose, the prodromal stage lasts from a few minutes to a few hours. The person suffers nervousness, confusion, nausea and vomiting, a loss of consciousness, and burning sensations of the skin. A latent period may last several hours. Manifest illness occurs five to six hours after exposure, resulting in diarrhea, convulsions, coma, and death.

Death caused by the CNS syndrome is not fully understood. CNS damage may result from damage to the blood vessels that supply the system, thus causing **edema** (swelling) in the cranial vault, **vasculitis** (inflammation of blood vessels), and **meningitis** (inflammation of the spinal cord and brain membranes). It is thought that death is caused by increased pressure in the cranial vault as a result of elevated fluid content from the previously mentioned changes.

Even though the hematopoietic and GI syndromes are taking place, the person does not live long enough to exhibit these syndromes.

LOCAL TISSUE DAMAGE

All organs and body tissues can be affected by partial body irradiation. The result is death to some of the cells, which results in **atrophy** (shrinking) of the tissue or organ. This in turn may lead to that organ or tissue becoming nonfunctional, or to recovery. With high enough doses, any local tissue will react. Tissue response depends on its radiosensitivity, reproduction, and maturation rates. The skin, gonads, and extremities are examples of local tissues that can be affected.

Skin

Because of the early uses of radiation and radiation therapy, the skin is the tissue that we have a good deal of data about. During the early years of radiology, because of the low X-ray tube potentials, unshielded X-ray tubes, and long exposure times, many people suffered **inflammation**, erythema, and **desquamation** (peeling) to their skin. X–ray-induced erythema was possibly the first observed biological response to irradiation. Radiation-induced skin erythema is analogous to that seen after extended exposure to the sun.

The skin is composed of an outer layer (**epidermis**), a middle layer of connective tissue (**dermis**), and a **subcutaneous** layer of fat and connective tissue. Accessory structures in the skin that originate in the dermis include the hair **follicles** (sac), **sebaceous** (oily secretion) glands, sweat glands, and sensory receptors. All the skin's cell layers and accessory structures are involved in the response to irradiation. Figure 4–4 illustrates the skin and accessory structures.

The epidermis is composed of cell layers that consist of both mature nondividing cells (surface cells) and immature dividing cells (basal layer cells). The skin's surface regularly loses cells that must be replaced by the basal layer cells, at the rate of approximately 2% per day. The characteristics of the epidermis basal cells thus make the skin radiosensitive.

Notes:

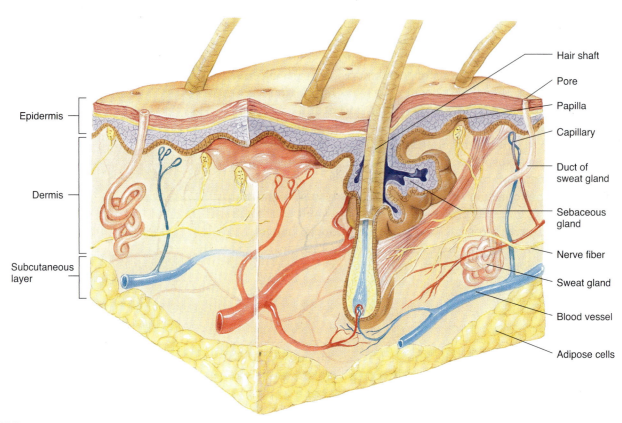

Epidermis

Dermis

Subcutaneous
layer

Hair shaft

Pore

Papilla

Capillary

Duct of
sweat gland

Sebaceous
gland

Nerve fiber

Sweat gland

Blood vessel

Adipose cells

FIGURE 4–4
Skin

Notes:

Within one to two days of a single dose of 100 to 1,000 rad, the skin may exhibit mild erythema. This initial erythema is followed by a more severe erythema in about two weeks. Prior to the introduction of radiation units, the **skin erythema dose (SED)** was used as a measure of the amount of radiation a person had received. Using data from people who were irradiated superficially with therapeutic X-rays, the skin erythema dose necessary to affect 50% of people so irradiated **(SED50)** is estimated to be approximately 600 rad (6 Gy). Skin erythema is considered to follow a nonlinear, threshold dose-response relationship.

When the epidermis is exposed to moderate doses, it is permitted to heal by regenerating, which results in insignificant late changes. However, when exposed to high doses, late changes including atrophy, fibrosis, changes in pigmentation, ulcers, **necrosis** (tissue death), and cancer may occur.

Since hair follicles are actively growing tissue, they are radiosensitive. Moderate doses may cause temporary epilation or **alopecia** (hair loss), with high doses possibly resulting in permanent epilation.

Sebaceous and sweat glands are considered to be relatively **radioresistant**. Exposure to high doses causes glandular atrophy and fibrosis that result in minimal or no function.

Subjecting the skin to chronic irradiation may result in nonmalignant changes. The early radiologists developed hands and forearms that were calloused, discolored, and weathered in appearance. Their skin became tight and brittle, which led to cracking and flaking.

Because of the use of intensifying screens, beam-restricting devices, and radiation protection guidelines, today's doses from diagnostic radiographic and fluoroscopic exams pose minimal hazard in regard to the previously mentioned changes. Table 4–3 summarizes the effects of radiation on skin.

Notes: _____

TABLE 4–3

Radiation Effects on Skin

Spectrum of Effects on Skin

Early Effects	Late Effects	Effect on Accessory Structures
Erythema	Atrophy	Epilation
Inflammation Dry Desquamation Moist desquamation	Fibrosis Hyper-/hypo-pigmentation Ulceration Necrosis Cancer	Destruction of sweat and sebaceous glands

Dose/Time—Response Relationship

Dose	Radiation Dose Area	Exposure Internal	Type of Reaction or Damage
<1 Gy (100 rads)	Small	Short	No visible effect
2–6 Gy (200–600 rads)	Small	Short	Erythema in 1–2 days after exposure; persists until day 5–6; reappears on day 10–12; maximum on day 18–20; persists until day 30–40. Temporary hair loss if >3 Gy (300 rads).
6–10 Gy (600–1,000 rads)	Small	Short	More serious erythema caused by damage of basal cells. Symptoms appear earlier, are more intense, and healing is delayed.
15 Gy (1,500 rads) or 30 Gy (3,000 rads)	Small Small	Short <4 weeks	Severe erythema, followed by dry desquamation and delayed/incomplete healing.
20–50 Gy (2,000–5,000 rads) or 40 Gy (4,000 rads)	Limited Limited	Short <4 weeks	Intense erythema, acute radiation dermatitis with moist desquamation, edema, dermal hypoplasia, vascular damage, and permanent hair loss, permanent tanning, destruction of sweat glands, vascular damage. If >5 Gy (5,000 rads) followed by ulceration/necrosis.
20 Gy (2,000 rads)	Hands or other small area	Several years small daily doses (1–2 rads)	No early or intermediate changes. Late changes manifested by dry cracked skin, nails curled and cracked, intractable ulcers, possible cancerous changes.

(Reproduced with permission from Bushberg, J. T., Seibert, J. A., Leidholt, E. M., & Boone, J. M. [2001]. *The essential physics of medical imaging* [2nd ed.]. Philadelphia: Lippincott, Williams and Wilkins.)

Notes:

Eyes

The lens of the eye contains radiosensitive cells that may be damaged or even destroyed by radiation. Because the body is not able to naturally remove damaged cells, they may accumulate to the point of causing cataracts. The formation of cataracts caused by radiation is termed **radiation cataractogenesis**. The extent of opacity and chance of occurrence are proportional to the dose.

Radiation-induced cataracts follow a threshold, nonlinear dose-response relationship. The threshold dose is thought to be approximately 200 rad (2 Gy). At doses of greater than 700 rad (7 Gy), all people irradiated will develop cataracts. The average latent period for cataract formation is approximately 15 years. High LET radiation has a high RBE for cataractogenesis by a factor of two or more. The efficiency of cataractogenesis is decreased by exposure to chronic doses.

Cataractogenesis was common among early radiation personnel and patients because of the extremely high doses from long exposure times and from exposures being produced by equipment that was poorly shielded. Cataractogenesis among today's radiation personnel is rare. It is nearly impossible for today's radiation personnel to reach the threshold dose. As the highest exposures to the eyes are received during fluoroscopic examinations, it is suggested that protective eyewear be worn while working in this high-dose area. Protective lens shields should be provided to patients as long as their use does not interfere with the exam.

Gonads

Human gonads are extremely radiosensitive. Doses as low as 10 rad have caused observable responses. As gonads create germ cells that control fertility and heredity, their response to irradiation has been analyzed thoroughly.

Much of the data regarding gonadal irradiation response has come from animal experiments, and some has come from radiation therapy patients, radiation accident victims, and experiments on volunteer convicts.

The male testes and the female ovaries react differently to radiation because of variations in the way their germ cells progress from the stem cell phase to the mature cell. Figure 4–5 contrasts the life cycle of the **oogonia** with that of **spermatogonia**.

Both the ovaries and testes produce germ cells, but they have different rates and times in regard to the way they develop from **stem cell** to mature cell. The ovary stem cells, the oogonia, multiply only during fetal life. During midpregnancy, the oogonia in the fetus number about seven million, and then start to decline in number throughout life. Conversely, the stem cells of the testes, the spermatogonia, are constantly reproducing.

Male With the exception of the testes, the majority of the male gonad tissue is radioresistant. The testes contain the mature spermatozoa, which are nondividing, differentiated, and radioresistant; they

Male:

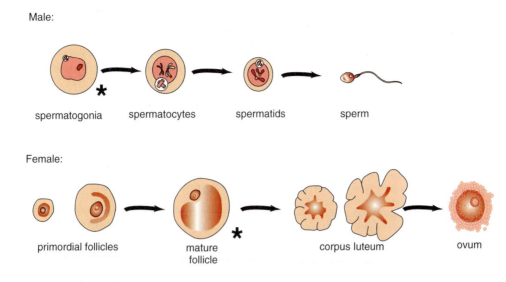

spermatogonia   spermatocytes   spermatids   sperm

Female:

primordial follicles   mature follicle   corpus luteum   ovum

* most radiosensitive

FIGURE 4–5
Oogonia vs. spermatogonia life cycle

also include the immature spermatogonia, which are rapidly dividing, undifferentiated, and radiosensitive. The main effect of radiation on the male gonads is damage to and reduction in the number of the spermatogonia, which ultimately leads to depletion of mature sperm, a process called **maturation depletion**. After testicular irradiation, there is a variable period of fertility caused by the radioresistance of the mature sperm. Depending on the dose, this period of fertility is followed by either temporary or permanent sterility. The cause of sterility is from the loss of immature spermatogonia that divide and replace the mature sperm lost from the testes. A dose of 200 to 250 rads produces temporary sterility, which may last up to one year. An acute dose of 500 to 600 rads causes permanent sterility.

Besides the possibility of sterility, another danger of irradiating the testes is the production of chromosomal abnormalities that may be passed on to future generations. The previously mentioned fertile period that occurs post-exposure does not eliminate the chance of damage to the chromosomes in the functional spermatozoa. Also, chromosome damage to the immature spermatogonia cannot be ruled out.

Diagnostic radiology consists of acute low doses to patients and chronic low doses to personnel that present no danger regarding sterility. Nevertheless, these doses may cause chromosomal abnormalities that could result in mutations in future generations. Because of this, the testes should be shielded from unnecessary radiation whenever practical.

Female   The ova, which are enclosed within the follicles, are specified by size as small, intermediate, and large. The radiosensitivity of the ova is as follows: most sensitive = intermediate follicles; most resistant = small follicles; and moderately sensitive = mature follicles. The ova do not continuously divide and replace those that

Notes:

are lost during menstruation. During ovulation, an ovum is released from a mature follicle. This is followed by either fertilization or menstruation. Following moderate doses of radiation to the ovaries, there is an initial period of fertility. This is caused by the presence of moderately resistant mature follicles that can release an ovum. The fertile period is succeeded by either temporary or permanent sterility. These sterilities are from the ova receiving damage in the radiosensitive intermediate follicles, which restricts their maturation and release.

A dose of 10 rads can restrain and retard menstruation. Sterility is a function of age, with the fetus and child being particularly radiosensitive. There is a decline in sensitivity until approximately age 30, when sensitivity begins to increase continually with age. Doses of 200 rads produce temporary sterility. An acute dose of approximately 500 to 600 rads will cause permanent sterility.

There is anxiety about the chance of genetic changes in the functional ova after being irradiated. Even though fertility recurs after low to moderate doses, it may be possible that the functional ova have suffered chromosomal damage, which may produce abnormal offspring or even nonvisible mutations that will not become manifest until future generations.

Analogous to the male, because of the acute low doses received by patients and chronic low doses received by personnel, the likelihood of female sterility is minimal. However, as mentioned previously, the possibility of chromosomal damage cannot be excluded. Therefore, the ovaries should be shielded from radiation whenever practical.

HEMATOLOGIC EFFECTS

In the 1920s and 1930s, periodic blood examinations were used to monitor radiology personnel. Included in these exams were total cell and white cell differential counts. We now know that it takes a minimum whole-body dose of about 25 rads (250 mGy) to cause hematologic depression. Based on current radiation protection standards, we now know that these people were heavily irradiated. Periodic blood examinations for radiation protection purposes are not justified for current radiation protection programs.

Hemopoietic System

The hemopoietic system includes bone marrow, circulating blood, lymph nodes, spleen, and thymus.

Included in bone marrow tissues are the parenchymal cells of the marrow, which include stem cells for cells in circulating blood and fat cells, and connective tissue **stroma** (support tissue). The two types of marrow found in adults are red and yellow. Red marrow, which includes a large number of stem cells along with fat cells, supplies mature functional cells to circulating blood. In the adult this marrow is located in the ribs, ends of long bones, vertebrae, sternum, and skull. Yellow marrow, composed mostly of fat cells with few stem cells, does not actively deliver mature cells to the circulating blood. Because of its fat content, the yellow marrow is also known as fatty marrow.

In contrast to an adult, whose bone marrow is found in definite sites, there is uniform distribution of bone marrow in the fetus. Also, the majority of fetal bone marrow is red bone marrow.

The principal response of bone marrow to radiation is a decrease in the number of stem cells. Low radiation doses cause a slight decrease in stem cells followed by recovery within a few weeks post-exposure. With moderate and high doses the depletion of stem cells is more intense, which leads either to a longer recovery period and/or less recovery. Less recovery is exhibited as an increased number of fat and connective tissue, and a permanent decrease of stem cells.

Even though all bone marrow stem cells are considered to be highly radiosensitive, the different cells display diversity as to their radiosensitivity. The most sensitive stem cells are the **erythroblasts** (precursor cells for red blood cells). Next in sensitivity are the **myelocytes** (precursors for white blood cells). The least sensitive stem cells are the **megakaryocytes** (precursors for platelets). Exposure to low radiation doses causes decreased stem cell numbers with rapid recovery. Moderate to high doses result in a more intense decrease in all cell lines accompanied by either slow or incomplete recovery of cell numbers.

Except for lymphocytes, cells in the circulating blood are considered radioresistant. Nevertheless, the circulating blood is an indication of how much damage the bone marrow has received. If there is a decrease in the number of stem cells in the marrow, there will be a coinciding decrease in the number of mature circulating cells.

The coincidence of damage to the bone marrow in the circulating blood cells depends on: a) the sensitivity of the various stem cells and b) the life span of each cell line. All circulating blood cells have a limited life span, which varies on the average from 1 day (**granulocytes**) to 120 days (erythrocytes).

Following radiation exposure, the lymphocytes are the first cells to be reduced (doses as low as 10 rads will decrease count). Second to respond are the neutrophils (doses of 50 rads are required to cause decrease). Last to respond are the platelets and red blood cells (doses greater than 50 rads are necessary). Figure 4–6 illustrates typical hematologic depression following bone marrow doses of (a) 100 rads and (b) 300 rads.

Low doses to the lymphocytes cause a minimal depression, which is followed by recovery and a return to pre-exposure lymphocyte values. After a moderate dose the lymphocyte counts approach zero within a few days, followed by full recovery within a few months post-exposure.

Within one week post-exposure, the neutrophil count falls to minimal values. Recovery begins shortly thereafter and within one month post-exposure, neutrophil counts approach normal.

For platelets and red blood cells, low doses in the moderate range have negligible effects. Higher doses in the moderate range cause

Notes:

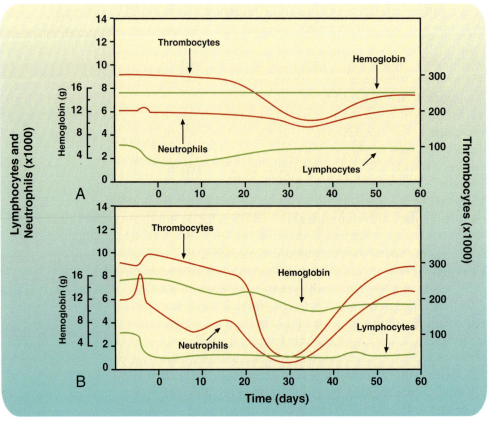

FIGURE 4–6

Hematologic depression bone marrow doses (Adapted from Andrews, G. [1980]. Medical management of accidental total-body irradiation. In *The medical basis for radiation accident preparedness*. K. F. Hubner, & S. A. Fry [eds.]. New York: Elsevier.)

Notes:

obvious cell depression. For these cells, recovery begins four weeks post-exposure, and usually is complete in a few months.

If there is a decrease in the numbers of these various cells, there may be consequences throughout life. The body's defense mechanisms rely on neutrophils and lymphocytes in fighting off infections. If these cells are depleted, the person will be more vulnerable to infection. Platelets are required for blood clotting. If these cells are depleted, there is increased chance for hemorrhage. If there is depression of red blood cells, the result will be anemia.

Regarding decreased cell counts, diagnostic dose ranges present no significant dangers to the blood and blood-forming organs of patients or occupationally exposed personnel, although there have been chromosomal changes observed in this dose range.

CYTOGENETIC EFFECTS

Chromosomal damage can occur with low and high radiation doses. Although structural changes may be caused by either direct or indirect action, the majority of chromosomal damage occurs from indirect ionization. Damage results in breakage of the chromosome.

The structural changes to the chromosome that occur after irradiation are called **aberrations** (imperfection), **lesions**, or **anomalies** (departure from normal). Chromosome aberrations that are caused by radiation can take place in both genetic and somatic cells. If chromosomal aberrations are not repaired before DNA synthesis, these aberrations may be transmitted during mitosis and meiosis.

Radiation-induced chromosomal damage that occurs before DNA synthesis is known as chromosomal aberration. If chromosomal repair does not happen before the S-phase of the cell cycle, a chromosomal break will be replicated. With chromosomal aberrations, both daughter cells inherit a damaged chromatid.

Radiation-induced chromosomal damage that occurs after DNA synthesis is called a chromatid aberration. While in the S-phase of the cell cycle, a chromosome duplicates itself. The two analogous chromosomes that are produced are known as sister chromatids. If only one pair of chromatids is damaged, only one daughter cell will be affected.

A chromatid aberration occurs after DNA synthesis. During the DNA synthesis phase, a chromosome duplicates itself. The two analogous chromosomes created are called sister chromatids. If only one pair of chromatids is injured, only one daughter cell will be affected.

The two primary types of chromosomal aberrations include single-break and double-break damage.

With single-break damage, a part of a chromosome arm is broken off. If the broken piece does not reattach itself, this is termed a terminal deletion; if it inverts and then reattaches itself, it is termed an inversion; if it attaches itself to a different chromosome, it is termed duplication.

In double-break damage, two portions of the chromosome are broken off. If the two broken pieces do not reattach themselves, this is termed interstitial deletion; if the broken pieces invert and reattach themselves to the chromosome arm, this is termed inversion; if one or both pieces attach to a different chromosome, this is termed duplication; with translocation, two chromosomes exchange pieces.

Factors that influence the repair of chromosomal aberrations include the stage of cell cycle and the type and location of the aberrations. The broken ends of chromosomes exhibit a strong force of cohesion. Recombination of chromosomes occurs in methods that produce aberrations such as **acentrics** (on the outside), **dicentrics** (having two centers), and rings. Figure 4–7 depicts common chromosomal aberrations and consequences.

The magnitude of total genetic damage that is transmitted by chromosomal aberrations depends upon the cell type, number and kind of genes damaged, and whether or not the aberration occurred in somatic or genetic cells.

If there is a change in a chromosome, there are corresponding changes in DNA. These changes in DNA cause the genetic information in the cell to be altered. This change in genetic information is called a mutation.

Notes:

	Breakage	Recombination	Replication	Anaphasic Separation
A. One break in one chromosome		NONE		
B. Two breaks in one chromosome Rings				or
C. One break in two chromosomes Translocation				
D. One break in two chromosomes Dicentrics				

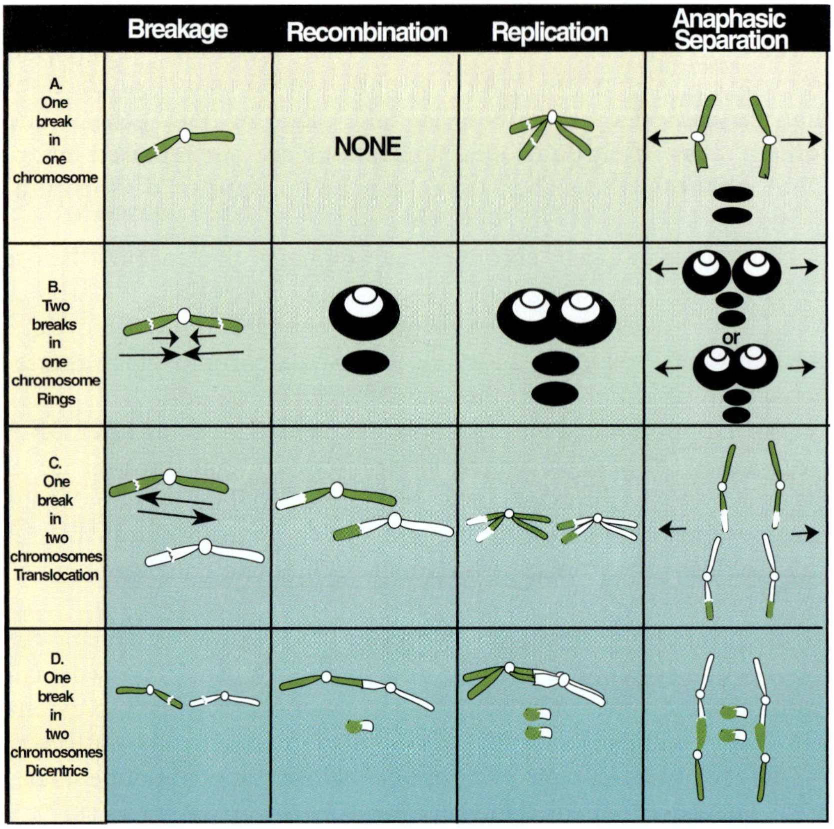

FIGURE 4–7

Common chromosome aberrations and consequences (Reproduced with permission from Bushberg, J. T., Seibert, J. A., Leidholt, E. M., & Boone, J. M. [2001]. *The essential physics of medical imaging* [2nd ed.]. Philadelphia: Lippincott, Williams and Wilkins.)

A **karyotype**, which is a chromosome map, is used for cytogenetic analysis of chromosomes. Photographs (photomicrographs) are taken and enlarged of the cell nucleus during metaphase that demonstrate each chromosome separately. The individual chromosomes are cut out and paired with their sister chromosomes on the map.

Consequences of chromosomal aberrations may not be able to be determined. If there is cell death, this is obviously a significant result. Numerous cell mutations go undetected and do not cause cell death. These discrete cell changes may be critical to humans. **Somatic** mutations have consequences for only that person. Genetic mutations can affect reproductive organs or the parent's **gametes**, which may affect future generations. It is presumed that genetic effects are cumulative.

Radiation cytogenetic data have shown that practically all types of chromosomal aberrations may be caused by radiation. The rate of production of aberrations is related to both total radiation dose and dose rate, and these appear to be nonthreshold. Chromosomal aberrations may be caused by both low and high radiation doses. Radiation effects on chromosomes appear to be nonspecific and are not desirable.

KEY CONCEPTS

- Hematologic syndrome is exhibited by destruction of bone marrow caused by a reduction in production of red and white blood cells and platelets resulting from radiation exposure. Death may occur as a result of anemia and infection. Gastrointestinal syndrome is exhibited by nausea, vomiting, cramps, and diarrhea as a result of damage to the villi in the small intestine, which leads to a lack of absorption. Dehydration and infection are the results. Central nervous system syndrome is exhibited by nervousness, confusion, nausea, vomiting, loss of consciousness, and burning sensations of the skin, which are the result of damage to blood vessels and increased intracranial pressure.

- Local tissue damage to the skin results in inflammation, redness, and a breakdown of the tissue layers. Higher doses of radiation cause hair loss, changes in pigmentation, ulcers, tissue death, and cancer. Radiation damage to the eyes results in cataracts. Tissue damage to the reproductive system as a result of radiation exposure may result in immature reproductive cell death leading to infertility and the possibility of genetic mutations in offspring.

- Radiation effects on the hematologic system reduce the number of stem cells produced by the bone marrow. A decrease in the number of white and red blood cells, as well as platelets, also occurs. Cytogenic effects as a result of radiation exposure result in damage and mutation of chromosomes.

American Society of Radiologic Technologists

CURRICULUM

The material presented in this chapter reflects the following area(s) of the ASRT Curriculum Guide:

Topic:

Radiation Biology

Content:

  III. Radiation Effects

  IV. Radiosensitivity and Response

Topic:

Radiation Protection

Content:

  II. Units, Detection, and Measurement

Notes:

CHAPTER

REVIEW QUESTIONS & EXERCISES
Crossword Puzzle

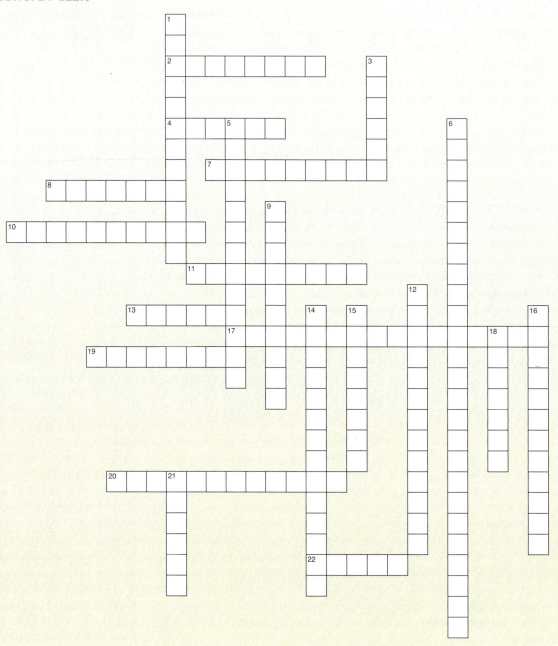

Across

2. On the outside.

4. The second stage in the response to radiation exposure in which changes are taking place within the body system that may either result in death or recovery.

7. Depression of all blood cell counts.

8. Shrinking.

10. Precursors for white blood cells.

11. Oily secretion.

13. Reduction in red blood cell counts.

17. A measure of the amount of radiation a person received.

19. The third stage in the response to radiation exposure in which body systems show signs and symptoms of exposure.

20. Redness and swelling at site of exposure.

22. Swelling.

Down

1. Red blood cells with a life cycle of one day.

3. Supportive tissue of an organism.

5. Precursors for red blood cells.

6. Formation of cataracts caused by exposure to radiation.

9. Inflammation of blood vessels.

12. Reproductive cells of the male.

14. Precursors for platelets.

15. The relationship of signs and symptoms to a specific disease or trauma.

16. Peeling skin.

18. Reproductive cells of the female.

21. Lethal dose to kill 50% of a population in 60 days.

Matching

Match the definition in the right column with the correct term from the left column.

_____ 1. Aberration

_____ 2. Alopecia

_____ 3. Anomaly

_____ 4. Crypts of Lieberkuhn

_____ 5. Dermis

_____ 6. Dicentric

_____ 7. Epidermis

_____ 8. Follicles

_____ 9. Hemopoietic

_____ 10. Karyotype

_____ 11. LD50/30

_____ 12. Lesion

_____ 13. Maturation depletion

_____ 14. Meningitis

_____ 15. Necrosis

_____ 16. Prodromal

_____ 17. Radioresistant

_____ 18. SED50

_____ 19. Somatic

_____ 20. Stem cell

_____ 21. Subcutaneous

_____ 22. Threshold dose

a. Imperfection
b. Open wound
c. Radiosensitive cells that are a precursor to the population of villi cells
d. Immature cells
e. Radiation dose necessary to affect 50% of a population
f. Departure from normal
g. The dose at which symptoms will occur
h. Pertaining to the development of blood cells
i. Having no reaction or ill effects of exposure to radiation
j. Chromosome map
k. The first stage in the response to radiation exposure
l. Hair loss
m. Middle layer of the skin
n. A chromosome that has two centers or two centromeres
o. Outer layer of the skin
p. Sacs or cavities
q. Inflammation of the membranes of the spinal cord and brain
r. Lethal dose to kill 50% of a population in 30 days
s. Tissue death
t. Reduction in the number of mature sperm
u. Nonreproductive cells
v. Inner layer of skin

Multiple Choice

1. A whole body radiation dose given in a period of seconds to minutes produces a clinical pattern called:
   a. mortality rate.
   b. relative biological effectiveness.
   c. acute radiation syndrome.
   d. clinical body dose.

2. A reddening of the skin cause by radiation damage is referred to as:
   a. epistaxis.
   b. epilation.
   c. cataractogenesis.
   d. erythema.

3. Which of the following would be considered an early response to irradiation?
   a. genetic damage
   b. leukemia
   c. life span shortening
   d. cytogenetic damage

4. Death from a single dose of whole body irradiation primarily involves damage to the:
   a. skin.
   b. bone marrow.
   c. skeletal system.
   d. respiratory system.

5. What is the principal response of the blood caused by radiation exposure?
   a. chromosome rearrangement
   b. chromosome fragmentation
   c. decrease in cell number
   d. cell proliferation stimulation

6. What is the approximate dose necessary to the ovaries to produce permanent sterility?
   a. 50 rad
   b. 100 rad
   c. 150 rad
   d. 200 rad

7. What is the approximate human SED50?
   a. 100 rad
   b. 300 rad
   c. 600 rad
   d. 1,000 rad

EXPLORING THE WEB

1. Search the Web for additional information on acute radiation syndromes. What resources are available? Create flash cards outlining the signs and symptoms of each syndrome for review and study.

   _____

   _____

   _____

   _____

2. Search the Web for examples of local tissue damage related to radiation exposure. What are you able to find on radiation exposure of skin, eyes, and gonads? How are females affected differently than males?

   _____

   _____

   _____

   _____

3. Search the Web for examples of chromosomal and cellular effects of radiation exposure. Can you find any case studies that illustrate these effects? What additional information can you find on the effects of radiation exposure on the hematologic system?

   _____

   _____

   _____

   _____

CASE STUDY

Your sibling tells you she saw a clip on YouTube about the radiation accident in Chernobyl. She asks you what is meant by the term acute radiation syndrome. Briefly describe this for her.

_____

_____

_____

_____

_____

_____

CHAPTER 5

Effects of Long-term Exposure to Radiation

KEY TERMS

Absolute risk model

Acute

Ankylosing spondylitis

BEIR

Benign

Carcinogenic

Carcinoma

Chronic

Doubling dose

Excess risk

Fibrosis

Follicular

Genetically significant dose (GSD)

Hypoxic

Leukemia

Loci

Lymphoid

Malignant

OBJECTIVES

Upon completion of this chapter, the reader should be able to:

- Discuss epidemiology
- Explain risk estimation models
- Examine radiation-induced malignancies
- Identify life-span shortening
- Discuss genetic damage
- Explain irradiation of the fetus
- Analyze stochastic and nonstochastic effects

Notes:

EPIDEMIOLOGY

Since the first documented case of radiation-induced **carcinoma** (growth or tumor) in 1902, it has been established that radiation is **carcinogenic** (cancer causing). Shortly after the discovery of X-rays, there were hundreds of cases of radiation-induced skin cancers reported by radiology personnel. It is now known that radiation is also responsible for causing other types of malignancies.

Although it has been well established that at high doses and high-dose rates radiation is carcinogenic, this is not the case with the low doses that are associated with occupational exposures. Predominately through animal and statistical studies of human population groups, radiation has been associated with causing cancer. Risks to low levels of exposure are small, but exactly how small is debatable.

TABLE 5–1

Sources of Data on Radiation Exposure to Humans

Atomic Bomb Detonation Exposures and Fallout
    Survivors
    Offspring of survivors

Medical Exposures
    Treatment of *tinea capitis*
    X-ray treatment of ankylosing spondylitis
    Prenatal diagnostic X-ray
    X-ray therapy for enlarged thymus glands
    Fluoroscopic guided pneumothorax for the treatment of tuberculosis
    Thorotrast (radioactive contrast material used in angiography 1925–1945)
    Treatment of neoplastic diseases (e.g., breast cancer, Wilms' tumor, cancer of the cervix, and leukemia)

Occupational Exposures
    Radium dial painters (1920s)
    Uranium miners and millers
    Nuclear dockyard workers
    Nuclear materials enrichment and processing workers
    Participants in nuclear weapons tests
    Construction workers
    Industrial photography workers
    Radioisotope production workers
    Reactor personnel
    Civil aviation and astronautic personnel
    Phosphate fertilizer industry workers
    Scientific researchers
    Diagnostic and therapeutic radiation medical personnel

Epidemiologic Comparisons of Areas with High Background
    Radiation

Reproduced with permission from Bushberg, J. T., Seibert, J. A., Leidholt, E. M., & Boone, J. M. (2001). *The essential physics of medical imaging* (2nd ed.). Philadelphia: Lippincott, Williams and Wilkins.

Incidence rates for radiation-induced cancer are determined by contrasting the expected occurrence in a control group (the general population) with the occurrence in an experimental group (the irradiated population). Risk factors are then calculated for the experimental group. The science that examines the incidence, distribution, and control of disease in a population is termed epidemiology.

The following populations are used as sources of data on the incidence of radiation-induced cancer:

1. Atomic bomb survivors
2. Medically exposed patients
3. Occupationally exposed personnel
4. Populations that receive high natural background exposure

Table 5–1 lists sources of data on radiation exposure to humans.

Limitations on epidemiologic studies include the following:

- Failure to control experimental group for other known carcinogens
- Insufficient observation periods that permit full demonstration of cancers with long latent periods
- Using improper control groups
- Deficient or incorrect health records

Table 5–2 summarizes some of the main epidemiologic studies from which current dose-response estimates are derived.

Figure 5–1 is a graphic representation of various radiation sources that contribute to the total average effective dose for persons living in the United States.

Dose-Response Curves

Dose-response curves have been created by scientists who predict cancer risks in human populations that have been exposed to low levels of ionizing radiation. These dose-response curves are non-threshold linear, linear quadratic, and quadratic. Figure 5–2 illustrates linear and linear quadratic dose-response curves.

Nonthreshold linear curves overestimate cancer incidence at lower doses from low LET radiation and accordingly are used for radiation protection guidelines when estimating the overall cancer risk from diagnostic and occupational exposures.

Relative vs. Absolute Risk

The relative or multiplicative risk model explains how age at the time of radiation exposure may influence the cancer risk estimate. This model theorizes that following the latent period, the excess risk is a multiple of the natural age-specific cancer risk for the population being studied.

Another theory is the **absolute** or additive **risk model**. This model estimates a continual increase in risk that is independent of

Notes:

TABLE 5–2

Dose-Response Epidemiologic Studies

Summary of Major Epidemiologic Investigations That Form the Basis of Current Cancer Dose-Response Estimates in Human Populations*

Population and Exposure	Effects Observed	Strengths and Limitations
Atomic Bomb Survivors: A mortality study of approximately 120,000 residents of Hiroshima and Nagasaki (1950) among whom 93,000 were exposed at the time of the bombing. This group continues to be followed. The latest mortality assessment through 1987 has been completed. New dose estimates have been made recently which determined that neutrons were not, as previously thought, a significant component of the dose for either of the two cities. Mean organ doses have been calculated for 12 organs. Approximately 20,000 received doses between 1–5 cGy (1–5 rads) while ~1,100 received doses in excess of 2 Gy (200 rads).	A total of 483 excess cancers are thought to have been induced by radiation exposure resulting in an excess cancer mortality of 205. The natural incidence for this population would have predicted 2,670 cancers. The number of expected, observed, and excess cancers by organ system is shown below. This data applies to the 41,000 persons who received 0.01 Sv (1 rem) or more. The mean dose was 0.23 Sv (23 rem). No statistically significant radiation-related increases were observed for uterine cancer, cervical cancer, pancreatic cancer, rectal cancer, multiple myeloma, non-Hodgkin's lymphoma, or chronic lymphocytic leukemia.	The analysis of the atom bomb survivors is the single most important cohort that influences current radiation-induced cancer risk estimates. The population is large and there is a wide range of doses from which it is possible to make determinations of the dose-response and the effects of modifying factors such as age on the induction of cancer. Data at high doses are limited; thus, the analysis included only individuals in whom the doses to internal organs were less than 4 Gy (400 rads). The survivors were not representative of a normal Japanese population in so far as many of the adult males were away on military service, while those remaining presumably had some physical condition preventing them from active service. In addition, children and the elderly perished shortly after the detonation in greater numbers than did young adults, suggesting the possibility that the survivors may represent a hardier subset of the population.

Cancer Type	Incidence Data		
	Expected	Observed	Excess
Breast	200	295	95
Lung	365	456	91
Stomach	1,222	1,307	85
Leukemia	67	141	74
Thyroid	94	132	38
Colon	194	223	29
Skin	76	98	22
Bladder	98	115	17
Liver	95	109	14
Esophagus	79	84	5
Brain & CNS	67	71	4
Bone & connective tissue	12	16	4
Non-Hodgkin's lymphoma	72	76	4
Multiple myeloma	29	30	1
TOTALS	2,670	3,153	483

TABLE 5–2 (continued)

Dose-Response Epidemiologic Studies

Summary of Major Epidemiologic Investigations That Form the Basis of Current Cancer Dose-Response Estimates in Human Populations*

Population and Exposure	Effects Observed	Strengths and Limitations
Ankylosing Spondylitis: This cohort consists of approximately 14,000 patients treated with radiotherapy to the spine for ankylosing spondylitis throughout the United Kingdom between 1935–1954. Although individual dose records were not available, estimates were made that ranged from 1–25 Gy (100–2,500 rads) to the bone marrow and other various organs.	Mortality has been reported through 1982, at which point 727 cancer deaths had been reported. Excess leukemia rates were reported from which all absolute risk of 0.8 excess cases/cGy (rad)/year per million was estimated.	This group represents one of the largest bodies of data on radiation-induced leukemia in humans for which fairly good dose estimates exist. Control groups were suboptimal, however, and doses were largely unfractionated. In addition, only cancer mortality (not incidence) was available for this cohort.
Postpartum Mastitis Study: This group consists of approximately 600 women, mostly between the ages of 20 and 40, treated with radiotherapy for postpartum acute mastitis in New York in the 1940s and 1950s for which ~1,200 non-exposed women with mastitis and siblings of both groups of women served as controls. Breast tissue doses ranged from 0.6–14 Gy (60–1,400 rad).	A 45-year follow-up identified excess breast cancer in this population as compared with the general female population of New York.	A legitimate objection to using the data from this study to establish radiation-induced breast cancer risk factors is the uncertainty as to what effect the inflammatory changes associated with postpartum mastitis and the hormonal changes due to pregnancy have on the risk of breast cancer.
Radium Dial Painters: Young women who ingested radium (Ra-226 and Ra-228 with half-lives of approximately 1,600 and 7 years, respectively) while licking their brushes (containing luminous radium sulfate) to a sharp point during the application of luminous paint on dials and clocks in the 1920s and 1930s. Over 800 followed.	Large increase in osteogenic sarcoma. Osteogenic sarcoma is a rare cancer (~5/106). Relative risk in the population was greater than 100 x's. No increase was seen below doses of 5 Gy (500 rad) but rose sharply thereafter.	This is one of only a few studies that analyzed the radiocarcinogenic effectiveness of internal contamination with high LET radiation in humans.
Thorotrast: Several populations were studied in which individuals were injected intravascularly with an X-ray contrast media, Thorotrast, used between 1925–1945. Thorotrast contains 25% by weight radioactive colloidal Th-232 dioxide. Th-232 is an alpha emitter with a half-life of approximately 14 billion years.	Particles were deposited in the reticuloendothelial systems. Noted increase in number of liver cancers, particularly angiosarcomas, bile duct carcinomas, and hepatic cell carcinomas. Evaluation of the data resulted in estimates of alpha radiation-induced liver cancer risk of approximately 300/104 per Gy (100 rad), which appears to be linear with dose.	Dose estimates are fairly good. However, the extent to which the chemical toxicity of the Thorotrast may have influenced the risk is not known.

*Adapted from the 1990 National Academy of Sciences/National Research Council Committee on the Biological Effects of Ionizing Radiation report entitled, *The Health Effects of Exposure to Low Levels of Ionizing Radiation (BEIR V).*

Sources of Radiation Exposure to the US Population

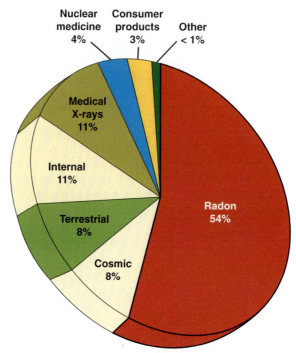

FIGURE 5–1
Sources of radiation exposure to U.S. populations

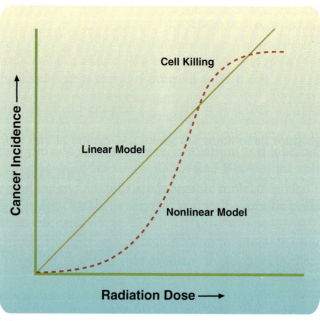

FIGURE 5–2
Linear and quadratic dose-response models

the spontaneous age-specific cancer risk at the time of exposure. Figure 5–3 compares the relative and absolute risk models.

It is speculated that as a person ages, his cancer risk increases. Figure 5–4 demonstrates the effect of age on incidence.

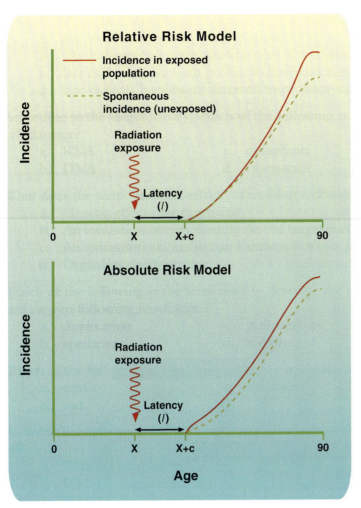

FIGURE 5–3
Relative and absolute risk models

Risk Expression   Relative risk is one method of expressing the risk from radiation to an exposed population. This risk is the ratio of cancer incidence in an exposed population to that of an unexposed population. It can be used when there is no exact knowledge of radiation dose.

$$\text{The formula for relative risk} = \frac{\text{observed cases}}{\text{expected cases}}$$

EXAMPLE

A relative risk of 1.5 would indicate a 50% increase in the irradiated group as compared with the non-irradiated group.

Relative risk rates range from 1 to 10, with 1 representing no risk at all. Most reports for the observed late effects in humans are in the range from 1 to 2.

Absolute risk states risk in terms of number of cases/106 persons/rad/year. This type of risk assumes a linear dose-response relationship. Absolute risk can be determined when at least two different dose levels are known.

Notes:

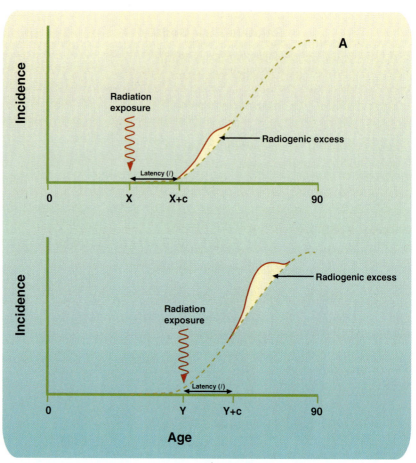

FIGURE 5–4
Effect of age on cancer incidence

EXAMPLE

A study of radiation-induced **leukemia** (cancer of blood-forming cells in bone marrow) was performed after diagnostic levels of radiation. Four hundred cases were observed in 150,000 people irradiated. The normal incidence of leukemia is 120 cases per 100,000. If the normal incidence were presumed to occur in a non-irradiated population, what is the relative risk of radiation-induced leukemia?

$$\text{Correct response: Relative risk} = \frac{\text{observed cases}}{\text{expected cases}}$$

$$\frac{400}{150,000} = 0.003 \qquad \frac{120}{100,000} = 0.0012$$

$$\text{Relative risk} = \frac{0.003}{0.0012} = 2.5$$

EXAMPLE

Absolute risk for radiation-induced breast cancer is presumed to be 6 cases/10⁶ persons/rad/yr at a 15-year at-risk period. If 10,000 women receive 1 rad during mammography, what would be the total number of cancers expected to be produced?

Correct response:

$$(6 \text{ cases}/10^6 \text{ persons/rad/year})(10^4 \text{ persons})(1 \text{ rad})(15 \text{ year}) = 0.9$$

$$\frac{6}{1,000,000} = 0.000006$$

$$0.000006 \times 10^4 \times 1 \times 15 = 0.9$$

Excess risk is another way to express risk. This risk is described as the number of excess cases observed compared with the expected spontaneous occurrence. When scientists can observe the number of cases in the irradiated population and compare this with the number that is normally expected, excess risk can be determined.

The formula for excess risk = observed cases − expected cases.

EXAMPLE

In a population of 2,000 radiologists, 13 cases of skin cancer were detected. The incidence for the general population is 0.5/100,000. How many excess skin cancers were produced in the radiologist population?

Correct response:

excess cases = observed cases − expected cases = 13 − 0.000005 = ~12.9

The relative and absolute risk models are most often used for expressing risk. The **BEIR** Committee (Committee on the Biological Effects of Ionizing Radiation), which is associated with the National Academy of Sciences, used the **relative risk model**.

Table 5–3 lists the overall risk and relative probabilities of radiation-induced cancer mortality in various organs for different age groups.

TABLE 5–3

Risk and Relative Probabilities of Cancer for Different Ages

Overall Risk and Relative Probabilities of Radiation-Induced Cancer Mortality in Various Organs for Different Age Groups[a]

Organ	Age Group		
	0–19 Years	0–90 Years	20–64 Years
Stomach	0.243	0.266	0.303
Lung	0.245	0.203	0.144
Bone Marrow	0.054	0.091	0.137
Bladder	0.030	0.054	0.081
Colon	0.218	0.154	0.078
Esophagus	0.023	0.040	0.062
Ovary[b]	0.011 (0.22)	0.017 (0.034)	0.024 (0.048)
Breast[b]	0.030 (0.60)	0.025 (0.05)	0.021 (0.042)
Remainder	0.150	0.150	0.150
Total	1.000	1.000	1.000
Risk 10^{-2}/Sv (10^{-4}/rem)	12	5.4	4

[a]Adapted from ICRP Report No. 60

[b]This table represents the ICRP's risk coefficients for a working population that is assumed to be half women and half men. The risks for ovaries and breasts for women alone (in parentheses) is therefore twice this risk. No coefficient was specifically given for testes, which is included in the remainder risk coefficient.

Notes:

RADIATION-INDUCED MALIGNANCIES

Many biological effects that are radiation-induced are discovered shortly after exposure. However, ionizing radiation is capable of causing damage that does not manifest itself for years or even decades.

Radiation-induced malignancies include leukemia, skin carcinoma, thyroid cancer, breast cancer, **osteosarcoma** (bone cancer), and lung cancer.

Leukemia

The first incidence of radiation-induced leukemia was in 1911. Since then, radiation has been associated with leukemia in studies of adult population groups that include atomic bomb survivors, **ankylosing spondylitis** (immobility of the vertebrae) patients who were treated with radiation, and radiologists.

Data from the atomic bomb survivors from Hiroshima and Nagasaki demonstrate a substantial increase in the incidence of leukemia when comparing the exposed with the unexposed population. From 1950–1956, 64 out of 117 new cases of leukemia were associated with radiation. In Hiroshima, 61 leukemia deaths were observed as compared with the expected incidence of 12.

$$\text{Relative risk} = \frac{\text{observed cases}}{\text{expected cases}} = \frac{61}{12} = 5.08$$

In Nagasaki, 20 leukemia deaths were observed as compared with the expected incidence of 7.

$$\text{Relative risk} = \frac{20}{7} = 2.85$$

Increased rates of leukemia were observed at Hiroshima at low doses (20–50 rads), but these increases were not seen at Nagasaki. These differences in incidence are attributed to the different types of radiation that each city was exposed to. Approximately 90% of the dose at Nagasaki was from X-rays, whereas at Hiroshima approximately half the dose was from X-rays and half was from neutrons. Neutrons have a higher RBE than X-rays, and are thus more biologically damaging.

From 1935 to 1944, approximately 15,000 patients with ankylosing spondylitis were treated with radiation in Great Britain. These patients received both acute and fractionated doses to the pelvis and spine that ranged from 100 to 2,000 R. A fractionated dose is one that is given in smaller quantities over a period of time.

In a two-year follow-up study, seven cases of leukemia were documented as compared with the expected incidence of one. In patients who received doses over 2,000 R, there was an increased incidence of leukemia of over 100%.

The early radiologists make up another group where radiation is considered to cause leukemia. A study in the United States of 425 radiologists who died between 1948 and 1961 shows an incidence of 12 cases of leukemia as compared with an expected incidence of 4.

A British study of radiologists who entered practice after 1921 demonstrated no excess in leukemia. This study is of significance because it contradicts the American radiologist study.

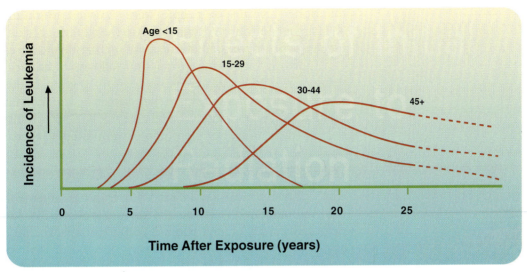

FIGURE 5–5
Effect of age at time of exposure (From Ichuimaru et al. [1976]. Incidence of leukemia in atomic bomb survivors, Hiroshima and Nagasaki, 1950–1971, by radiation dose years after exposure, age, and type of leukemia. *Technical Report RERF* 10–76. Hiroshima: Radiation Effects Research Foundation.)

Currently, the incidence of leukemia among American radiologists is not higher than other physician specialties. There is no evidence of radiation-induced leukemia in studies of American radiographers.

With the incidence of leukemia in the United States at approximately 70/10,000, it is considered a rare disease. Even so, leukemia is one of the most frequently observed radiation-induced cancers. It is responsible for approximately one-sixth of the fatalities from **radiocarcinogenesis**. Leukemia can be **acute** (rapid and severe) or **chronic** (slow and progressive). It may be either **lymphoid** (in lymph tissue) or **myeloid** (in marrow). Excluding chronic lymphocytic leukemia, irradiated human population groups and animals that have been irradiated experimentally show increases in all forms of leukemia.

Age at the time of irradiation influences the incidence of leukemia. The incidence of radiation-induced leukemia decreases with age, as does the interval of increased risk. Figure 5–5 illustrates the effect of age at time of exposure on incidence of leukemia.

Radiation-induced leukemia is judged to be linear and nonthreshold, and has a latent period of 4 to 7 years with an at-risk period of 15 to 20 years.

The BEIR committee suggests a relative risk, nonlinear dose-response relationship for leukemia. It estimates the excess lifetime risk to be 10/10,000 (0.1%) after an exposure of 10 rads (0.1 Gy).

Skin Carcinoma

Within 15 years of the discovery of X-rays, hundreds of cases of skin carcinoma were reported by radiology personnel. Also occurring during the early years of radiation is another source of data from people who were treated with radiation for acne and ringworm and developed skin cancer years later.

Even though radiation-induced skin carcinomas cannot be distinguished from skin carcinomas caused by other methods, there is enough proof to connect radiation with skin cancer. The previously

Notes:

mentioned groups of people were exposed to unfiltered low kV X-rays that deliver very high doses to the superficial skin layers. These incidents prompted radiation safety regulations to be established.

Radiation-induced skin carcinoma follows a threshold dose-response relationship and has a latent period of 5 to 10 years. In the 500 to 2,000 rad range, the relative risk for skin cancer is 4 to 1. With doses in the 6,000 to 10,000 rad range, the relative risk is 27 to 1. Radiation-induced skin carcinomas are not present in current radiology personnel.

Thyroid Cancer

The 1920s and 1930s saw infants with thymic enlargement being treated with radiotherapy. Doses to the thyroid were in the 120 to 6,000 R range. In a study of approximately 3,000 infants who received on average 120 rads, there were 24 observed cases of thyroid cancer. The expected incidence was 0.24 cases. This resulted in a hundredfold increase in thyroid cancer incidence. In a control group composed of approximately 5,000 unexposed infants, no cases of thyroid cancer were demonstrated. Another source of data comes from the offspring of the Marshall Islanders who were accidentally exposed to fallout radiation from nuclear bomb testing. These children in later years demonstrated an increased incidence of all types of thyroid disease, which included **benign** (nonprogressive) and **malignant** (progressive) tumors.

Studies of individuals who were children at the time of the atomic bombings in Nagasaki and Hiroshima have also shown increased incidences of thyroid cancer.

Thyroid cancer is responsible for approximately 12% of the deaths attributed to radiation-induced malignancies. Females have approximately a three to five times greater risk for radiation-induced thyroid cancer than males, because of hormonal influences on thyroid function.

Radiation-induced thyroid cancers are either **papillary** (nipple-like protrusion) or **follicular** (cavity), which are usually benign and slow growing, with a mortality rate of about 5%. The latent period for benign nodules is 5 to 35 years, and for malignant nodules 10 to 35 years. Internal irradiations from radionuclides such as iodine-131 have not been proven to cause thyroid cancer. The dose-response relationships for thyroid cancers are linear, nonthreshold.

Breast Cancer

The United States' breast cancer incidence for women is approximately 85/100,000 year or 1 in 11 lifetime. With low LET radiation, breast cancer risk seems to be age dependent. The risk for the 15-year-old age group (30/10,000 or 0.3% year) is approximately 50 times higher after an exposure of 10 rads (0.1 Gy) than in women over the age of 55. According to the BEIR report, risk estimates for women in the 25-, 35-, and 45-year-old age groups are 0.05, 0.04, and 0.02%, respectively. Breast cancer data appear to fit a linear dose-response relationship. In order to double the natural incidence of breast cancer, a dose of approximately 80 rads (0.8 Gy) is necessary. According to data from current acute and chronic exposure studies, it seems that fractionating the dose reduces the risk of low LET radiation-induced breast cancer. The latent period varies from 10 to 40 years. Absolute risk is estimated to be approximately six cases/106 persons/rad/year.

Because of recent improvements in mammography, there have been significant reductions in breast radiation doses. Even though theoretically mammography could increase the risk of breast cancer, studies have not demonstrated that the low doses received during a mammogram increase the risk of breast cancer.

Osteosarcoma

Bone cancers were noted in the watch-dial painters in the early 1920s. These people applied luminescent **radium** on watch hands and faces. In order to get a fine tip on their brush, they would put the tip in their mouth and pull it out. Radium was ingested by these workers and, being metabolically similar to calcium, was deposited in bone. Radium has a half-life of 1,620 years, meaning that it continued to be deposited at full strength throughout the person's lifetime. In a 1978 study of approximately 1,500 women employed in the industry before 1930, there were 61 cases of bone cancer, and 21 cases of sinus and mastoid carcinomas. Data analysis of the painters indicated an overall relative risk of 122:1. The absolute risk is 0.11 cases/106 persons/rad/year. Osteosarcoma follows a linear quadratic dose-response relationship.

Lung Cancer

Increased incidences of lung cancer have been demonstrated in miners of uranium and pitchblende. Data from studies of the German pitchblende miners revealed that approximately 50% of them died from lung carcinoma. The general population had negligible incidences of lung cancer. These carcinomas were attributed to the radiation exposure received from **radon** in the mines.

A study of uranium miners in the Colorado plateau from 1950 to 1967 demonstrated 62 cases of lung cancer, which is six times the expected number. One of the decay products of uranium is the gas radon. The miners would inhale the radon, which would be deposited in their lungs. It would then decay into a stable isotope of lead. During decay, alpha-particles, which are high LET and therefore high RBE, were released and resulted in high local doses.

Dose-response relationships for radiation-induced lung cancer are linear nonthreshold. Based on data from over 4,000 uranium miners, an absolute risk of 1.3 cases/106 persons/rad/year has been calculated.

Table 5–4 lists the spontaneous incidence and sensitivity of various tissues to radiation-induced cancer.

LIFE-SPAN SHORTENING

Data from studies of animals that received acute and chronic radiation indicate that animals that were chronically irradiated died younger than animals that were not irradiated. Examinations of the dead animals showed a decreased number of **parenchymal** (essential, life-sustaining) cells and blood vessels along with increases in

Notes:

TABLE 5–4

Spontaneous Incidence and Sensitivity of Tissues to Cancer

Spontaneous Incidence and Sensitivity of Various Tissues to Radiation-Induced Cancer[a]

Site or Type of Cancer	Spontaneous Incidence	Radiation Sensitivity
Most Frequent Radiation-Induced Cancers		
Female breast	Very high	High
Thyroid	Low	Very high, especially in females
Lung (bronchus)	Very high	Moderate
Leukemia	Moderate	Very high
Alimentary tract	High	Moderate to low
Less Frequent Radiation-Induced Cancers		
Pharynx	Low	Moderate
Liver and biliary tract	Low	Moderate
Pancreas	Moderate	Moderate
Lymphomas	Moderate	Moderate
Kidney and bladder	Moderate	Low
Brain and nervous system	Low	Low
Salivary glands	Very low	Low
Bone	Very low	Low
Skin	High	Low
Magnitude of Radiation Risk Uncertain		
Larynx	Moderate	Low
Nasal sinuses	Very low	Low
Parathyroid	Very low	Low
Ovary	Moderate	Low
Connective tissue	Very low	Low
Radiation Risk Not Demonstrated		
Prostate	Very high	Absent?
Uterus	Very high	Absent?
Testis	Low	Absent?
Mesothelium	Very low	Absent?
Chronic lymphatic leukemia	Low	Absent?

[a]Adapted from Committee on Radiological Units, Standards and Protection: *Medical Radiation: A Guide to Good Practice.* Chicago: American College of Radiology, 1985.

connective tissue in organs. These are suggestions of an aging process. This is regarded as radiation-induced aging. The correlation between life-span shortening and dose is linear, nonthreshold.

Nonspecific life-span shortening caused by radiation has been reported in humans, although it appears to be caused by other radiation-induced effects, for example, leukemia, especially in the low dose ranges.

Radiologists from the 1930s were found to die five years younger than a control group of other doctors. A repeat study in the 1960s showed that this difference in death had shrunk to zero. This may be credited to improved radiation protection guidelines.

Life-span shortening has not been observed in atomic bomb survivors, watch-dial painters, or X-ray patients. Data from radiographers in WWII also showed no such effects.

GENETIC DAMAGE

Evidence of the ability of ionizing radiation to produce genetic damage was first acquired from a comprehensive study of fruit flies done in 1927 by Herman Muller. Muller exposed male and female fruit flies to various doses of radiation, observed lethality and changes in appearance in offspring of irradiated parents, and compared these results with the unirradiated control group.

Muller's study concluded that:

1. No new or unique mutations are produced by radiation. Radiation simply increased the number of mutations found spontaneously in nature.
2. In the dose range of 25–400 R, the frequency of mutations was linear with dose. No threshold was observed. Equal dose increases were followed by an equal number of increases in the number of mutations. The observed effects were considered linear nonthreshold.
3. The majority of radiation-induced mutations were recessive. Both parents would have to carry the gene for an effect to be observed in offspring.
4. There were no dose rate or dose fractionation effects. This implies that mutations were single-hit and cumulative.

An ongoing experiment with irradiating mice was started by Russell in 1946. Data from this study demonstrate that:

1. Radiation is a powerful mutagenic agent.
2. The majority of mutations are unhealthy to the organism.
3. There are no unique mutations produced by radiation.
4. Radiation-induced genetic damage can occur as the result of a single mutation.

Initially, it was hypothesized that genetic effects were thought to be the most serious biological outcome from ionizing radiation. For the doses used in occupational and medical exposure, risks are small when compared with the spontaneous incidence of genetic aberrations, and are second to its carcinogenic capability.

Notes:

Epidemiologic studies have not demonstrated radiation-induced genetic effects, although mutations of human cells in culture have been shown. For given exposures, mutation rates found in the offspring of irradiated humans are much lower than those previously identified in insect populations.

The largest human population studied is that of atomic bomb survivors and their offspring. A blood screening of 27,000 children of atomic bomb survivors for 28 specific protein **loci** demonstrated only two mutations that might be caused by radiation exposure of their parents.

Previous studies of atomic bomb survivors' **progeny** (offspring) were performed to determine if exposure to radiation caused an increase in sex-linked genes that would result in increased prenatal death of males or alteration of the gender birth ratio. The results of this study were negative. Irradiation to human testes has demonstrated an increase in incidence of translocations, although no additional chromosomal aberrations in atomic bomb survivors' progeny have been detected.

In order to evaluate the genetic influence of low doses to the whole population, the term **genetically significant dose (GSD)** is used. The GSD is an average calculated from the gonadal dose received by the entire population. It takes into account the expected contribution of these people to children in future generations. The GSD assumes that this dose, if received by every member of the population, would have the identical genetic effect as the doses that are received by those people who are actually exposed to radiation. When determining the GSD, the equivalent dose to the gonads of each irradiated person is weighted for the number of offspring expected for a person of that sex and age.

The annual GSD from all radiation sources is approximately 130 mrem (1.3 mSv). The single largest contribution, approximately 102 mrem (1.02 mSv) or 78%, comes from natural background radiation, primarily from cosmic rays, terrestrial exposure, and radionuclides within the body. The contribution from radon is minimal at approximately 10 mrem (100 mSv).

Technological sources contribute to the GSD predominately in the form of medical exposures, approximately 20 mrem (200 mSv) or 15%. About two-thirds of this is attributable to irradiation of females and one-third to males. Exposure is higher for females because of the location of the ovaries within the pelvis, which places them in the primary beam during radiographs of the abdomen and pelvis. Table 5–5 lists the annual GSD in the U.S. population.

Data from experiments have given rise to the concept of the **doubling dose.** This is the dose of radiation required per generation to double the spontaneous mutation rate. The spontaneous mutation rate is approximately 6%.

EXAMPLE

If 5% of the progeny in each generation have mutations, the doubling dose would eventually cause 10% mutations.

In data extrapolated from animal studies, the doubling dose for humans is estimated to be in the range of 50 to 250 rads (0.5 and

TABLE 5–5

Annual GSD in the United States Population

Source	Contribution to GSD (mrem)	% of total
Natural Sources		
Radionuclides in body	36	
Terrestrial	28	
Cosmic	27	
Radon	10	
Cosmogenic	1	
Subtotal	102	78
Technological Sources		
Diagnostic X-rays	20	
Nuclear medicine	2	
Consumer products	5	
Other	< 1	
Subtotal	~ 28	22
Total	130	100

Notes:

2.5 Gy) for each generation. A dose range is given because of the differences in frequency of mutations that are observed with chronic and acute exposure. The doubling dose for chronic exposure tends to be toward the higher dose range, and for acute exposure is toward the lower end of the range.

Essentially, if each individual of childbearing potential in the entire population were exposed to a gonadal dose of 50–250 R for many generations, there would eventually be twice the number of mutations in their progeny.

It is estimated by the BEIR Committee that an exposure of 1 rad (1 cGy) given to the present generation would cause 6 to 65 additional genetic disorders per million births in the succeeding generation. If the population is continually exposed to an increased dose of 1 rad for each generation, equilibrium is created between the initiation of new genetic disorders and the loss of remaining ones. An additional 100 genetic disorders would be expected in the population at equilibrium, mostly from clinically mild autosomal dominant mutations. Chromosomal damage and recessive mutations contribute only minimally to the equilibrium rate. Even though some cancers are genetic in origin, it has not been proven that radiation has the capability to influence the inheritance of cancer susceptibility. Table 5–6 lists estimates of excess genetic effects following doses of 1 rad per generation.

TABLE 5–6

Estimates of Excess Genetic Effects Following Doses of 1 Rad Per Generation[a,b]

Typer of Disorder	Current Incidence per 10⁶ Live-Born Offspring	Additional Cases per 10⁶ Live-Born Offspring per 10 mSv per Generation	
		First Generation	Equilibrium
Autosomal dominant[c]			
Clinically severe	2,500	5–20	25
Clinically mild	7,500[d]	1–15	75
X–linked	400	<1	<5
Recessive	2,500	<1	VSI
Chromosomal			
Unbalanced translocations	600[e]	<5	VLI
Trisomies	3,800[f]	<1	<1
Congenital abnormalities	20,000–30,000	10	10–100
Other disorders of complex etiology[g]			
Heart disease	600,000	NE	NE
Cancer	300,000	NE	NE
Selected others	300,000	NE	NE

[a]Adapted from the 1990 National Academy of Sciences/National Research Council Committee on the Biological Effects of Ionizing Radiation report entitled, *The Health Effects of Exposure to Low Levels of Ionizing Radiation (BEIR V)*.

[b]Risks pertain to average population exposure of 10 mSv per generation to a population with the spontaneous genetic burden in humans and a doubling dose for chronic exposure of 1 Sv (100 rem). VSI = very slow increase; VLI = very little increase; NE = not estimated.

[c]"Clinically severe" assumes that survival and reproduction are reduced by 20–80% relative to normal. "Clinically mild" assumes that survival and reproduction are reduced by 1 to 20% relative to normal.

[d]Obtained by subtracting an estimated 2,500 clinically severe dominant traits from an estimated total incidence of dominant traits of 10,000.

[e]Estimated frequency from UNSCEAR Reports (1982 and 1986).

[f]Most frequent result of chromosomal nondisjunction among live-born children. Estimated frequency from UNSCEAR (1982 and 1986).

[g]Lifetime prevalence estimates may vary according to diagnostic criteria and other factors. The values given for heart disease and cancer are round-numbered approximations for all varieties of the diseases. With regard to heart disease, no implication is made that any form of heart disease is caused by radiation among exposed individuals. The effect, if any, results from mutations that may be induced by radiation and expressed in later generations, which contribute, along with other genes, to the genetic component of susceptibility. This is analogous to environmental risk factors that contribute to the environmental component of susceptibility. The magnitude of the genetic component in susceptibility to heart disease and other disorders with complex etiologies is unknown.

Notes:

The human gene pool has the ability to absorb large amounts of radiation damage without seriously affecting the population. Variations in natural background exposure do not contribute greatly to the population's genetic risk.

EXAMPLE

A dose of 10 rads (10 cGy) produces approximately only 200 additional genetic disorders/million live births in the first generation (0.002%/rad). The normal incidence of genetic disorders is approximately 1 in 20 or 5%. Therefore, the 10 rad (10 cGy) dose would cause an increase in the spontaneous rate of genetic disorders of less than 0.4%.

The doses associated with diagnostic and occupational radiation exposures, even though increasing the dose to the gonads of those irradiated, would not be anticipated to cause any significant risk to their offspring.

IRRADIATION OF THE FETUS

A developing organism is a highly dynamic system that is characterized by rapid cell proliferation, migration, and differentiation. Based upon the law of Bergonie and Tribondeau, we know that the developing embryo is very radiosensitive. The embryo's response to irradiation depends upon the following factors:

- total dose
- rate of dose
- quality of radiation
- stage of development

The combination of these factors determines the type and extent of damage that can occur. The principal effects of irradiation to the fetus include:

- prenatal or neonatal death
- congenital abnormalities
- growth impairment
- reduced intelligence
- genetic abnormalities
- cancer induction

A fetus undergoes three stages of development: pre-implantation, major organogenesis, and fetal or growth stage. Each of these stages is distinguished by differing responses to irradiation, which are caused by the relative radiosensitivity of the tissues at the time of exposure.

Data on the effects of irradiation *in utero* have been obtained from the offspring of the atomic bomb survivors and children whose mothers received diagnostic and therapeutic irradiation during pregnancy. Microcephaly and mental and growth retardation were the principal effects that were seen. Abnormalities of the eyes, genitals, and skeleton occurred less often.

Children from Hiroshima and Nagasaki who were irradiated *in utero* between the 8- to 25-week postconception period demonstrated lower IQ scores than did the non-irradiated children. These effects were not observed in those children who were exposed before week 8 or after week 25. This decrease in IQ was dependent on dose, and had a presumed threshold below 25 rads (250 mGy). These data demonstrated the greatest sensitivity for radiation-induced mental retardation is between 8 and 25 weeks, during which the risk is about 1/250 or 0.4% per 100 rad to the fetus.

Children who were irradiated *in utero* at the time of the atomic bomb detonation were observed to have microcephaly. The normal incidence of microcephaly is approximately 3%. In the dose range of

10–49 rads (100–490 mGy), the incidence of microcephaly was approximately 19% and 6% for the first and second trimesters, respectively. At doses greater than 100 rads (1 Gy) the microcephaly incidence jumped to approximately 83% and 42% for exposures in the first and second trimesters, respectively.

The predominant scientific opinion is that there are thresholds for the majority of congenital abnormalities. Compared with the spontaneous incidence of congenital anomalies, which is approximately 4–6%, doses less than 10 rads (100 mGy) carry negligible risk. At doses below this threshold, therapeutic abortions would not normally be warranted. Radiation was once used to induce therapeutic abortion in cases where surgery was considered to be unwise. The normal treatment was 350–500 rads (3.5–5 Gy) given over two days, which usually resulted in fetal death within one month. In current diagnostic procedures, fetal irradiation rarely exceeds 5 rads (50 mGy). This dose range has not demonstrated any significant risk for congenital malformation or retarded growth.

Pre-implantation Stage

This stage originates with the joining of the sperm and egg, and continues through day 9 when the **zygote** becomes deposited in the intrauterine wall. During this stage, the fertilized ovum is repeatedly dividing to form a ball of highly undifferentiated cells.

Radiation damage during this stage can cause prenatal death. The incidence of congenital abnormalities is low during this stage, although not completely absent. Embryos that survive display the all-or-nothing response. If prenatal death does not happen, visible signs of abnormalities are unlikely, as injured cells are repaired or replaced.

Factors that contribute to the cell's resistance to radiation-induced abnormalities include their capability of repair, undifferentiation, and the **hypoxic** (poorly oxygenated) state of the embryo. During the first few cell divisions, the cells are undifferentiated and are not predetermined for a specific organ system. Nevertheless, if there is chromosomal damage at this point, it may be passed on and expressed at a later time. Once cells are no longer indeterminate, losing even a few cells may cause anomalies, retarded growth, or prenatal death. The most critical times of exposure are at 12 hours postconception, when the two pronuclei fuse to the one-cell stage, and at 30 and 60 hours, which is when the first two divisions take place.

Radiation-induced chromosomal aberrations at the one-cell stage may lead to a loss of a chromosome in future cell divisions that would be similar throughout the embryo. At this early stage, the majority of chromosomal loss is fatal. If there is a loss of a sex chromosome in the female, this may cause **Turner's syndrome.** This syndrome is an endocrine disorder caused by failure of the ovaries to respond to pituitary hormone stimulation.

Data obtained from animal experiments show an increase in the spontaneous abortion rate after doses of 5–10 rads (50–100 mGy) given during the pre-implantation stage. Following implantation, doses of at least 25 rads (250 mGy) are necessary to cause prenatal death. The natural occurrence of spontaneous abortion is approximately 25–50%.

Major Organogenesis
The incidence of congenital abnormalities is more frequent during the period of major organogenesis, which is the second to eighth week after conception. The differentiation of cells to form specific organ systems occurs on a specific gestational day.

> **EXAMPLE**
>
> The stem cells of the CNS, the **neuroblasts,** appear on gestational day 18, the forebrain and eyes start to form on day 20, and primitive germ cells appear on day 21.

Organ systems are not at equal risk during the entire stage of major organogenesis. The critical period for probability of a malformation occurs when there is irradiation during the period of peak differentiation of that system. Some aberrations have demonstrated more than one critical period.

> **EXAMPLE**
>
> In mice, cataractogenesis has three critical periods.

Figure 5–6 demonstrates the critical periods for radiation-induced birth defects in humans.

Notes:

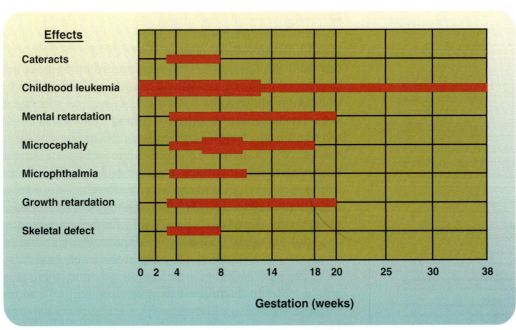

FIGURE 5–6

Critical periods for radiation-induced birth effects (Data from Dekaban, A. S. [1968]. Abnormalities in children exposed to x-irradiation during various stages of gestation: Tentative timetable of radiation injury to human fetus. *J Nucl Med, 9,* 471–477.)

The CNS is the only organ system that has shown a relationship between congenital anomalies and low LET radiation at doses less than 25 rads (250 mGy). Because of the depletion of cells, embryos that are irradiated early in organogenesis show the greatest intrauterine retardation of growth. Hiroshima atomic bomb survivors who received *in utero* exposures greater than 10 rads (100 mGy) showed increased incidences of microcephaly.

Overall, radiation-induced teratogenic effects are less frequent in humans than in animals. This is because of the smaller fraction of the gestational period in which humans are in organogenesis (for example, approximately 1/15 for humans vs. 1/3 for mice). However, the development of the CNS takes place over a much longer gestational period in humans than in animals, so it is more likely to be a target for radiation-induced injury. The CNS is not fully developed until approximately age 12 years. All cases of human irradiation *in utero* that resulted in gross malformations have been accompanied by CNS aberrations and/or retarded growth.

Each organ is unique in how it responds to the induction of radiation-induced malformations. Factors such as gestational age, radiation quality/quantity/dose rate, and oxygen tension, the type of cell undergoing differentiation, and how it relates to the surrounding tissues will influence the result.

Fetal Growth Stage

This stage starts following the end of major organogenesis (day 45) and continues until term. The incidence of radiation-induced prenatal death and congenital aberrations during this stage is negligible. The main radiation-induced anomalies seen during this stage involve the nervous system and sense organs. This corresponds with their relative growth and development. Damage caused during this stage may not manifest itself until later in life, for example, behavioral changes, reduced IQ, or cancer.

Cancer Risk *in Utero*
In data obtained by Stewart in 1956 in a retrospective study of childhood cancer in Great Britain referred to as the "Oxford Survey of Childhood Cancers," a correlation was seen between childhood leukemia and solid tumors and irradiation *in utero*. Similar studies have confirmed this observation, reporting a relative risk of approximately 1.4 for childhood cancer. This effect was not seen in the survivors of the atomic bomb who were irradiated *in utero*. These positive studies are widely disputed based on factors that include the influence of pre-existing medical conditions for which the exam was required and the lack of good estimates of fetal doses.

Human data have been examined by numerous national and international organizations that then developed risk estimates for carcinogenesis following *in utero* irradiation. **Neoplasms** are estimated to be up to three times more frequent following irradiation in the first trimester as compared to the second and third trimesters. Peak occurrence of childhood leukemia was between the ages of 2 and 4 and was higher in males. An increased risk of childhood leukemia continued through the 10th year of life, compared to the

14th year for solid tumors, the majority of which were neoplasms of the CNS. The current estimates for leukemia mortality are 2–3/10,000 after 1 rad (1 cGy) of low LET radiation. Solid tumors occur at approximately the same incidence. This brings the combined mortality from *in utero* irradiation to approximately 4–6/10,000 per rad (1 cGy). These mortality figures are thought to be identical to those cancers that occur spontaneously and in insufficient numbers to be easily identified in an exposed population.

In comparison, the natural total risk of mortality from malignancy through age 10 is 1/1200. If a fetus received a dose from a chest X-ray of 60 mrads (0.6 mGy), the chance of developing a fatal cancer during childhood from that exposure would be less than 1 in 27 million. The current effective dose equivalent limit to the fetus is no more than 500 mrem (5 mSv) during the gestational period, provided that the dose rate does not exceed 50 mrem (0.5 mSv) in any one month. If the maximum allowable dose was received, the chance of developing a fatal cancer during childhood from the exposure would be less than 1 in 3,300. While it is true that radiation exposure should be kept to a minimum, the risk at levels associated with occupational and diagnostic exposures is negligible when compared with other potential hazards.

Table 5–7 lists the effect of risk factors on pregnancy outcome.

TABLE 5–7

Effect of Risk Factors on Pregnancy Outcome[a]

Effect	Number Occurring from Natural Causes	Risk Factor	Excess Occurrences from Risk Factors
Radiation Risks			
Childhood Cancer			
Cancer death in children	1.4/1,000	Radiation dose of 1,000 mrems received before birth	0.6/1,000
Abnormalities			
		Radiation dose of 1,000 mrads received during specific periods after conception:	
Small head size	40/1,000	4–7 weeks > conception	5/1,000
Small head size	40/1,000	8–11 weeks > conception	9/1,000
Mental retardation	4/1,000	8–15 weeks > conception	4/1,000
Nonradiation Risks			
Occupation			
Stillbirth or spontaneous abortion	200/1,000	Work in high-risk occupation	90/1,000

(continues)

TABLE 5–7 (continued)

Effect of Risk Factors on Pregnancy Outcome[a]

Effect	Number Occurring from Natural Causes	Risk Factor	Excess Occurrences from Risk Factors
	Alcohol Consumption		
Fetal alcohol syndrome	1–2/1,000	2–4 drinks/day	100/1,000
Fetal alcohol syndrome	1–2/1,000	More than 4 drinks/day	200/1,000
Fetal alcohol syndrome	1–2/1,000	Chronic alcoholic (> 10 drinks/day)	350/1,000
Perinatal infant death	23/1,000	Chronic alcoholic (> 10 drinks/day)	170/1,000
Smoking			
Perinatal infant death	23/1,000	Less than 1 pack/day	5/1,000
Perinatal infant death	23/1,000	One pack or more/day	10/1,000

[a]Source: U.S. Nuclear Regulatory Commission (NRC) Regulatory Guide 8.13, Rev. 2, *Instruction Concerning Prenatal Radiation Exposure.*

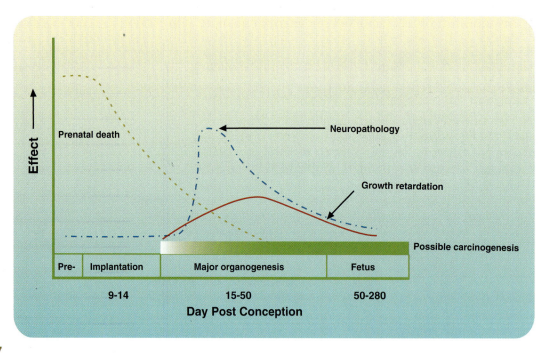

FIGURE 5–7

Relative incidence of radiation-induced health effects during stages of fetal development (Adapted from Mettler, F. A., & Moseley, R. D. [1985]. *Medical effects of ionizing radiation.* New York: Grune & Stratton.)

Notes:

Figure 5–7 depicts the relative incidence of radiation-induced health effects during the different stages of fetal development.

In utero irradiation risk can be put into perspective by examining the probability of birthing a healthy child after a given dose to the conceptus. Please refer to Table 5–8.

A fetal dose of even 1 rem (10 mSv) does not seriously affect the risks that are associated with pregnancy. Although therapeutic abortions

TABLE 5–8

Probability of Healthy Child after Given Dose to Conceptus

	Probability of Birthing Healthy Children[a]		
Dose[b] to Conceptus (mSv [mrem])	Child with No Malformation (Percentage)	Child Will Not Develop Cancer (Percentage)	Child Will Not Develop Cancer or Have a Malformation (Percentage)
0(0)	96	99.93	95.93
0.5(50)	95.999	99.927	95.928
1.0(100)	95.998	99.921	95.922
2.5(250)	95.995	99.908	95.91
5.0(500)	95.99	99.89	95.88
10.00(1000)	95.98	99.84	95.83

[a]From Wagner L. K., Hayman L. A.: Pregnancy in women radiologists. *Radiology*, 145:599–562, 1982.

[b]Refers to absorbed dose above natural background. This table assumes conservative risk estimates, and it is possible that there is no added risk.

because of fetal doses are rarely justified, each case should be analyzed individually and the risks explained to the patient. All efforts should be taken to reduce irradiation to the patient and especially the fetus. In looking at the relatively minute risk that is associated with diagnostic examinations, the postponement of clinically indicated examinations or scheduling examinations around the patient's menstrual cycle to avoid irradiation of a potential fetus are usually not warranted. Nevertheless, prior to diagnostic examinations that involve ionizing radiation, all fertile female patients should be questioned as to whether there is the possibility that they might be pregnant. If it is known that the patient is pregnant and alternative diagnostic procedures are not appropriate, the risks and benefits of the examination should be discussed with the patient prior to the examination.

STOCHASTIC AND NONSTOCHASTIC EFFECTS

The biological effects of irradiation are classified as either **stochastic** or **nonstochastic** (deterministic). Stochastic effects occur randomly in nature. Also referred to as the statistical response, a stochastic effect is one in which the probability of occurrence of effects, rather than their severity, increases with dose.

EXAMPLE

The chance of radiation-induced leukemia is considerably greater after an exposure to a dose at 100 rad (1 Gy) than at 1 rad (1 cGy), but there will be no difference in the severity of the disease if it occurs.

Stochastic effects are thought to be nonthreshold, as damage to a few cells or even a single cell could theoretically produce the disease. They are associated with the linear and linear quadratic dose-response curves. Therefore, even small exposures could carry some increased risk. Modern radiation protection programs are based on the assumption that risks are proportional to dose with no threshold. Stochastic effects are regarded as the main health risk from low-dose radiation from exposures in the diagnostic radiology department. Examples of stochastic effects include radiation-induced cancer and radiation-induced genetic effects.

If radiation exposure is high, the principal biological effects will be death of the cells caused by degenerative changes in the exposed tissue. If this is so, the severity of the injury, rather than its chance of occurring, increases with dose. These nonstochastic or deterministic effects are different from stochastic effects in that they need much higher doses to occur.

Nonstochastic or deterministic effects are thought to be threshold, as there are doses below which the effect is not observed. Examples of nonstochastic or deterministic effects from ionizing radiation are cataracts, erythema, **fibrosis,** and hematopoietic damage. Nonstochastic effects are relevant to serious radiation accidents, but are not likely to occur from diagnostic imaging examinations or routine occupational exposure. Nonstochastic or deterministic effects increase in severity with dose, and thus are considered to be threshold.

RADIATION HORMESIS

Radiation hormesis is the theory that ionizing radiation is benign at low levels of exposure, and that doses at the level of natural background radiation can be beneficial. This is in contrast to the linear no threshold model which posits that the negative health effects of ionizing radiation are proportional to the dose. The scientific consensus is not to accept radiation hormesis, despite a few papers to the contrary. The disagreement arises partly because very low doses of radiation have relatively small impacts on individual health outcomes. It is therefore difficult to detect the "signal" of decreased or increased morbidity and mortality due to low-level radiation exposure in the "noise" of other effects.

Radiation hormesis has been rejected by both the United States National Research Council (part of the National Academy of Sciences) and the National Council on Radiation Protection and Measurements (a body commissioned by the United States Congress).

KEY CONCEPTS

- The epidemiology of radiation exposure determines the incidence, distribution, and control of the disease in a particular population.

American Society of Radiologic Technologists

CURRICULUM

The material presented in this chapter reflects the following area(s) of the ASRT Curriculum Guide:

Topic:

Radiation Biology

Content:

III. Radiation Effects

IV. Radiosensitivity and Response

Topic:

Radiation Protection

Content:

II. Units, Detection, and Measurement

- Risk estimation models measure the amount of risk in a particular population at a particular point in time related to a particular disease.
- Cancer occurrences as a result of exposure to radiation are termed radiation-induced malignancies.
- Life-span shortening is the result of chronic exposure to radiation that results in the premature death of an individual.
- Genetic damage as a result of radiation is determined through the study of mutations in chromosomes and genetic coding that resulted from exposure of unborn children to radiation while *in utero*.
- The fetus will suffer adverse effects of irradiation while *in utero* at various growth stages. Cells that are undergoing rapid development upon exposure will show increased abnormalities and susceptibility to radiation-induced malignancies later in life.
- Stochastic effects occur randomly; the probability of being affected increases with the dose. Nonstochastic effects are deterministic; the severity of the injury increases with the dose, not the chance of it occurring.

Notes:

REVIEW QUESTIONS AND EXERCISES

Crossword Puzzle

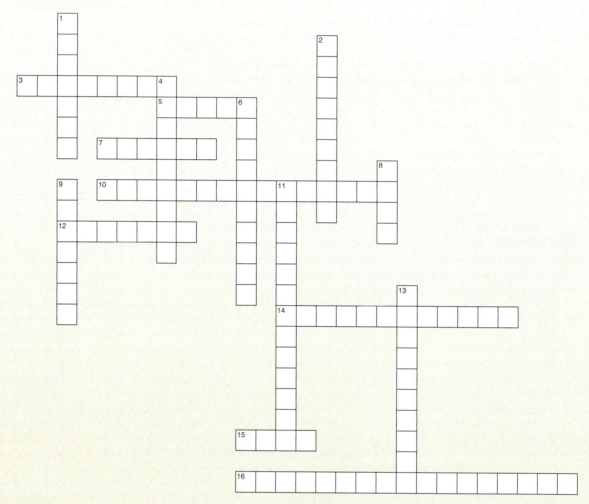

Across

3. Tumor.

5. Rapid, severe.

7. Radiogenic substance.

10. An endocrine disorder caused by the failure of the ovaries to respond to pituitary hormone stimulation.

12. Offspring.

14. Cancer-causing.

15. Spot, place of origin.

16. The ratio of cancer incidence in an exposed population to that of an unexposed population.

Down

1. Slow, progressive.

2. Nipple-like protrusion.

4. Progressive, threatening.

6. The number of excess cases of cancer observed compared with expected spontaneous occurrence.

8. Committee on the Biological Effects of Ionizing Radiation.

9. Low levels of oxygen.

11. Deterministic.

13. Cavity.

Matching

Match the term in the left column with the correct definition from the right column.

_____ **1.** Absolute risk model

_____ **2.** Ankylosing spondylitis

_____ **3.** Benign

_____ **4.** Carcinoma

_____ **5.** Doubling dose

_____ **6.** Fibrosis

_____ **7.** Genetically significant dose (GSD)

_____ **8.** Leukemia

_____ **9.** Lymphoid

_____ **10.** Myeloid

_____ **11.** Neuroblasts

_____ **12.** Osteosarcoma

_____ **13.** Parenchymal

_____ **14.** Radiocarcinogenesis

_____ **15.** Radon

_____ **16.** Stochastic

_____ **17.** Zygote

a. Marrow
b. Occurring randomly in nature
c. An average calculated from the gonadal dose received by the entire population and used to determine the genetic influence of low dose to whole population
d. Cancer of blood-forming cells in bone marrow
e. Essential life-sustaining cells
f. Radiation-producing cancer
g. Radiogenic gas
h. Estimates a continual increase in risk, independent of the age-specific cancer risk at time of exposure
i. A growth or tumor
j. The dose of radiation required per generation to double the spontaneous mutation rate
k. Nonprogressive
l. Bone cancer
m. Immobility of the vertebrae
n. Fertilized egg
o. Abnormal formation of fibrous tissue
p. Lymph tissue
q. Embryonic nerve cells

Multiple Choice

1. Epidemiology is defined as the study of:
   a. populations
   b. radiation
   c. physics
   d. statistics

2. The type of dose-response relationship demonstrated by human lethality is:
   a. linear, threshold
   b. nonlinear, threshold
   c. nonlinear, nonthreshold
   d. linear, nonthreshold

3. Which of the following is considered the most radiosensitive?
   a. fetus
   b. pediatric patient
   c. adult
   d. geriatric patient

4. What is the term that describes radiation damage that increases the probability of causing a late effect, but will not increase the severity of the effect?
   a. chronic
   b. congenital
   c. stochastic
   d. nonstochastic

5. What is the minimum radiation level below which no genetic or somatic damage would occur?

    a. 1 R   c. 10 R
    b. 5 R   d. no minimum level exists

6. Which of the following types of radiation-induced cancers demonstrates a threshold dose-response relationship?

    a. skin   c. lung
    b. bone   d. breast

7. Which of the following is most likely to follow irradiation *in utero* if the radiation is received during the organogenesis stage?

    a. prenatal death
    b. neonatal death
    c. latent malignancies
    d. congenital abnormalities

EXPLORING THE WEB

1. Search the Web for sites discussing the victims of Hiroshima, Nagaskai, and Chernobyl. What types of injury and mutation were discovered in these populations? What were the rates of morbidity and mortality in these areas?

    _____

    _____

    _____

    _____

2. Search the Web for additional information on risk models related to radiation exposure. Are there additional models that were not discussed in the text? How do they relate to what you have already learned? Can you find any case studies related to assessment of risk related to radiation exposure?

    _____

    _____

    _____

    _____

3. Search the Web for additional information on radiation-induced malignancies. What are the morbidity and mortality rates associated with each type of cancer found? Are incidences higher in males than in females?

    _____

    _____

    _____

    _____

CASE STUDY

You have performed an X-ray exam on a female who later determined she was pregnant at the time of the X-ray exposures. Discuss the factors that affect her embryo's response to radiation. Explain the possible principal effects of irradiation to her fetus.

_____
_____
_____
_____
_____
_____

SECTION 2 REVIEW

MULTIPLE CHOICE

1. A whole body radiation dose given in a period of seconds to minutes produces a clinical pattern called:
    a. mortality rate
    b. relative biological effectiveness
    c. acute radiation syndrome
    d. clinical body dose

2. When does the greatest radiation hazard to a fetus exist?
    a. first trimester
    b. second trimester
    c. third trimester
    d. unable to determine

3. A reddening of the skin caused by radiation damage is referred to as:
    a. epistaxis
    b. epilation
    c. erythema
    d. cataractogenesis

4. Which of the following is not an early response to irradiation?
    a. breast cancer
    b. skin erythema occurring 2 weeks post-exposure
    c. intestinal distress occurring 1 week post-exposure
    d. chromosome aberrations

5. The annual effective dose-equivalent limit for the fetus of an occupational worker is:
    a. 0.001 rem
    b. 0.01 rem
    c. 0.5 rem
    d. 1.0 rem

6. For humans, the LD50/30 is approximately:
    a. 50 rad
    b. 100 rad
    c. 200 rad
    d. 300 rad

7. Pertaining to irradiation of mammalian gonads:
    a. effects are independent of LET.
    b. for sterility, the dose-response relationship is linear, nonthreshold.
    c. in the male, the spermatocyte is more radiosensitive than the spermatogonia.
    d. depression of germ cells has been measured at doses as low as 10 rad.

8. The LD50/30 is representative of the dose:
    a. necessary to kill 10% of the cells in 50 days.
    b. necessary to kill 50% of the cells in 50 days.
    c. necessary to kill 50% of the cells in 30 days.
    d. necessary to kill 30% of the cells in 50 days.

9. Which of the following would be considered an early response to irradiation?
    a. genetic damage
    b. leukemia
    c. life-span shortening
    d. cytogenetic damage

10. The type of dose-response relationship demonstrated by human radiation lethality is:
    a. linear, threshold
    b. nonlinear, threshold
    c. nonlinear, nonthreshold
    d. linear, nonthreshold

11. What is the approximate dose necessary to the ovaries to produce permanent sterility?
    a. 50 rad
    b. 100 rad
    c. 150 rad
    d. 200 rad

12. Which acute radiation syndrome has a mean survival time that is independent of dose?
    a. hematologic
    b. gastrointestinal
    c. central nervous system
    d. unable to determine

13. What is the approximate human SED50?
    a. 100 rad
    b. 300 rad
    c. 600 rad
    d. 1000 rad

14. Which of the following is not an acute local tissue effect of radiation exposure?
    a. cataracts
    b. epilation
    c. temporary sterility
    d. skin erythema

15. Death from to a single dose of whole body irradiation primarily involves damage to the:
    a. skin
    b. bone marrow
    c. skeletal system
    d. respiratory system

16. What does "GSD" represent?
    a. general safe dose
    b. gonad safe dose
    c. germ safe dose
    d. genetically significant dose

17. What is the minimum radiation level below which no genetic or somatic damage would occur?
    a. 1 R
    b. 5 R
    c. 10 R
    d. no minimum level exists

18. What is the principal response of the blood caused by radiation exposure?
    a. chromosome rearrangement
    b. chromosome fragmentation
    c. decrease in cell number
    d. cell proliferation stimulation

19. Radiation cataractogenesis:
    a. follows a linear, nonthreshold dose-response relationship.
    b. follows a nonlinear, threshold dose-response relationship.
    c. exhibits a threshold of approximately 5 rad.
    d. has a latent period of 6 months.

20. Epidemiology is defined as the study of:
    a. populations.
    b. radiation.
    c. physics.
    d. statistics.

21. What is the approximate relative risk for development of radiation-induced leukemia?
    a. 0.1
    b. 0.5
    c. 1.0
    d. 1.5

22. The absolute risk factor for radiation-induced breast cancer is approximately _____ cases/10⁶/rad/year.
    a. 0.06
    b. 1.0
    c. 6
    d. 60

23. Radiation-induced lung cancer exhibits which of the following dose-response relationships?
    a. nonlinear, nonthreshold
    b. linear, nonthreshold
    c. linear, threshold
    d. nonlinear, threshold

24. What is the approximate latent period for radiation-induced leukemia?
    a. 6 months   c. 4 to 7 years
    b. 1 year   d. 20 years

25. Which of the following populations has not shown an increased incidence of radiation-induced leukemia?
    a. American radiographers
    b. American radiologists
    c. atomic bomb survivors
    d. radiotherapy patients

26. Which of the following types of radiation-induced cancers demonstrates a threshold dose-response relationship?
    a. skin   c. lung
    b. bone   d. breast

27. Which of the following is most likely after irradiation *in utero* if the radiation is received during the organogenesis stage?
    a. prenatal death   c. latent malignancies
    b. neonatal death   d. congenital abnormalities

28. What term describes radiation damage that increases the probability of causing a late effect but will not increase the severity of the effect?
    a. chronic   c. stochastic
    b. congenital   d. nonstochastic

29. Which of the following is the term used to describe the dose of radiation that will increase the number of mutations by a factor of two?
    a. doubling dose   c. nonstochastic dose
    b. stochastic dose   d. congenital dose

30. What is the approximate dose required to cause permanent male sterility?
    a. 5 rad   c. 250 rad
    b. 100 rad   d. 500 rad

31. Which of the following radiation syndromes would be caused by an acute whole-body exposure of 5,000 rad?
    a. hematologic syndrome
    b. gastrointestinal syndrome
    c. central nervous system syndrome
    d. unable to determine

32. Which of the following describes ulceration, necrosis, and loss of skin cells from irradiation?
    a. erythema   c. desquamation
    b. epilation   d. cataractogenesis

SECTION 3

Radiation Protection

A radiographer who is subjected to chronic low doses of radiation may be affected by its damaging effects if protection measures are not applied. The components and methods considered for minimizing patient exposure are also useful in reducing personnel exposure.

It is the responsibility of the radiographer to minimize ionizing radiation exposure to the patient. Even more essential is adoption of this responsibility into the everyday work habits and decision-making processes.

CHAPTER 6

Protection of Personnel

KEY TERMS

Agreement states

ALARA

Bone marrow dose

Controlled area

Cumulative timing device

Deadman type

Dose

Dosimetry

Early effect of radiation

Effective dose limit

Entrance skin exposure (ESE)

Film badge

Gonadal dose

Intermittent fluoroscopy

Inverse square law

Ionization chamber

OBJECTIVES

Upon completion of this chapter, the reader should be able to:

- Discuss the rationale for radiation protection
- Explain personnel monitors, dosimetry/monitor reports, and duties of the radiation safety officer
- Define and calculate the dose-limiting recommendations for diagnostic radiology personnel
- Explain structural shielding construction and list the items that influence this construction
- Describe how to decrease the radiographer's exposure during a mobile radiographic examination
- Identify ways to lessen the radiographer's exposure during a fluoroscopic examination
- Discuss how using distance can decrease radiation exposure
- Illustrate the inverse square law
- Identify protective garments that can be worn to reduce radiation exposure and explain when such garments should be used
- List the people and methods that can help with patient immobilization during an X-ray exposure

Notes:

RATIONALE FOR RADIATION PROTECTION

When humans are exposed to ionizing radiation, there is a risk of damage to their cells and offspring. The purpose of **radiation protection** is to lessen the likelihood of such occurrences. Figure 6–1 shows the sources of radiation exposure experienced in the United States.

If human cells respond to a high **dose** of radiation within minutes, days, or weeks after exposure, this is termed an **early effect of radiation**. The primary early effects to humans include hematologic depression, skin erythema, epilation, chromosome damage, gonad dysfunction, and death. In modern diagnostic radiology, doses of this quantity are not experienced.

If damage to human cells is not detected for months or years after radiation exposure, this is termed a **late effect of radiation**. The primary late effects to humans include radiation-induced cancer and genetic effects. Exposure to intermittent low doses of radiation over a long period of time is what we experience in modern diagnostic radiology.

Effective dose limits have been implemented to lessen the possibility of the occurrence of early and late effects of radiation.

MONITORING OF PERSONNEL

Because radiology personnel have the potential to be exposed to ionizing radiation, they must be monitored to ensure that their levels of exposure remain well below the annual dose-equivalent limits.

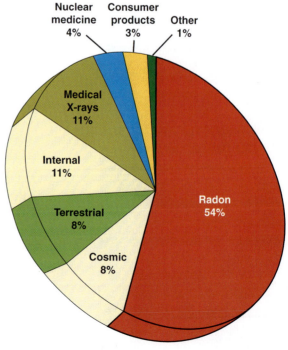

Sources of Radiation Exposure to the US Population

Nuclear medicine 4%
Consumer products 3%
Other 1%
Medical X-rays 11%
Internal 11%
Terrestrial 8%
Cosmic 8%
Radon 54%

FIGURE 6–1
Sources of radiation exposure

Monitoring of personnel is mandatory when they are likely to receive 10% of the annual effective dose-equivalent limit.

Measurement of ionizing radiation doses to personnel is termed **dosimetry. Personnel dosimeters** record external radiation doses. The types of personnel dosimeters used in diagnostic radiology include **film badges, thermoluminescent dosimeters (TLD), optically stimulated luminescence (OSL) dosimeters**, and **pocket dosimeters**. These devices are worn by radiology personnel during working hours. Film badges, OSLs, and TLDs are normally monitored monthly, and dosimetry reports are returned to the subscribing institution. This report documents the personnel's radiation dose equivalent for a specific month. The institution's radiation safety officer (RSO) reviews the monthly dosimetry report and posts it in an appropriate area. The RSO is responsible for seeing that personnel do not exceed occupational exposure limits.

Film Badges

Film badges are one type of personnel dosimeter (Figure 6–2). They measure occupational radiation exposure. Film badges consist of a small piece of special radiation-dosimetry film, similar to dental film, contained in a light-proof packet. This film packet is enclosed inside a plastic holder, which can be clipped to a person's clothing. The film packet is changed monthly. Metal filters composed of either copper or aluminum are placed inside the holder. These filters shield certain parts of the film that permit estimates of dosage and radiation energy. (Figure 6–3) Shallow and deep doses can be calculated according to the amount of darkening of the film after processing.

Film badges are usually worn at the collar level. If a lead apron is worn, the film badge must be worn at the collar level on the outside of the lead apron.

Film badges must be worn with the correct side of the badge facing forward. This allows the film badge company to determine whether the radiation dose received by the person came from in front of or from behind the wearer.

Companies who supply institutions with film badges provide a control badge, which is kept in a radiation-free area. It serves as a baseline when compared with the rest of the film badges after

Notes:

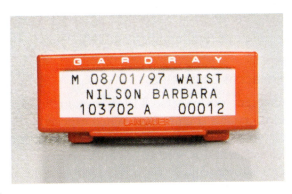

FIGURE 6–2

Film badge dosimeter (Courtesy of Landauer, Inc., Glenwood, IL)

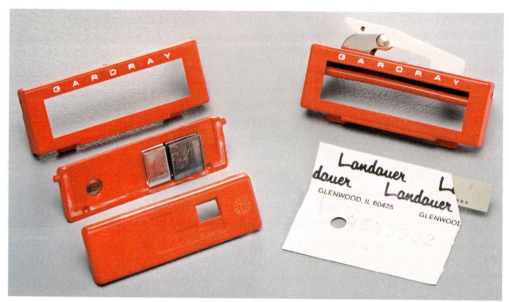

FIGURE 6–3
Film badge dosimeter inside view (Courtesy of Landauer, Inc., Glenwood, IL)

Notes:

processing by the monitoring company. After processing, the monitoring company constructs a characteristic curve similar to those used to determine film speed and contrast.

When personnel undergo medical and/or dental radiographs as a patient, the film badge should never be worn. Badges should be stored away from sources of radiation, and must be kept away from excessive heat and high humidity. They must be worn only for the designated period of time, and only by the person assigned to that badge.

Advantages of film badges:

- Simple to use
- Inexpensive
- Readily processed by commercial laboratories
- Provide a permanent record by laboratory and in radiology department

Disadvantages of film badges:

- Are not reusable
- Low limit of sensitivity (approximately 10 mrem)
- Accuracy limited to +/− 10–20%
- Susceptible to heat, humidity, and light leaks

Thermoluminescent Dosimeters

Thermoluminescent dosimeters (TLD) contain lithium fluoride or calcium fluoride crystals (Figure 6–4). When exposed to ionizing radiation, these crystals store radiant energy when heated. As they are heated, the crystals release energy as light, which is then measured by a machine that documents the radiation exposure based on how much light is emitted. There is a direct relationship between the intensity of light emitted and the radiation dose received by the crystals (Figure 6–5).

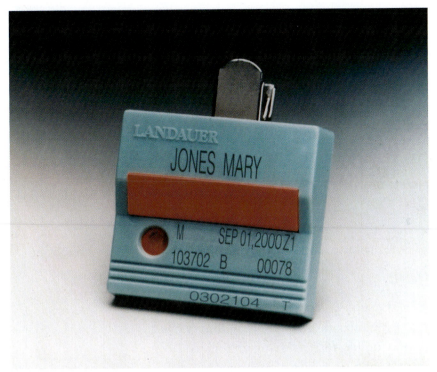

FIGURE 6–4
Thermoluminescent dosimeter (Courtesy of Landauer, Inc., Glenwood, IL)

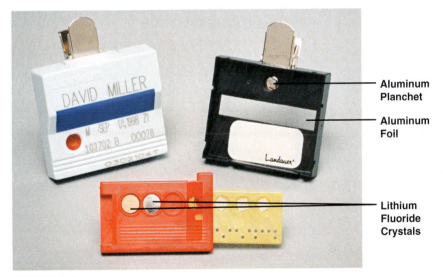

Aluminum
Planchet

Aluminum
Foil

Lithium
Fluoride
Crystals

FIGURE 6–5
Thermoluminescent dosimeter inside view (Courtesy of Landauer, Inc., Glenwood, IL)

TLDs are commonly worn as finger rings by nuclear medicine personnel to measure occupational exposure to their hands from handling radioisotopes (Figure 6–6).

Advantages of TLDs:

- Can be made very small
- Sealed in Teflon, minimizing chance of damage
- Low exposure limit, to 5 mrem
- Response to X-rays proportional up to approximately 400 R

Notes:

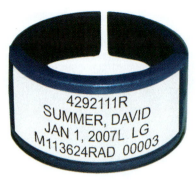

FIGURE 6–6
Ring dosimeter (Courtesy of Landauer, Inc., Glenwood, IL)

- Response almost independent of X-ray energy from about 50 kV to 50 mV
- Accuracy to approximately +/− 5%
- Response very similar to tissues
- Less sensitive to heat than film badge
- Can be worn as a ring on fingers
- Can be worn for three months
- Are reusable

Disadvantages of TLDs:

- Cannot be stored as a permanent record
- More expensive than film badge

Optically Stimulated Luminescence (OSL) Dosimeters

An optically stimulated luminescence (OSL) dosimeter contains filters composed of aluminum, tin, and copper. It also houses a thin strip of aluminum oxide (Figure 6–7). The strip is stimulated by

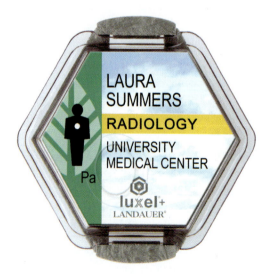

FIGURE 6–7
OSL dosimeter (Courtesy of Landauer, Inc., Glenwood, IL)

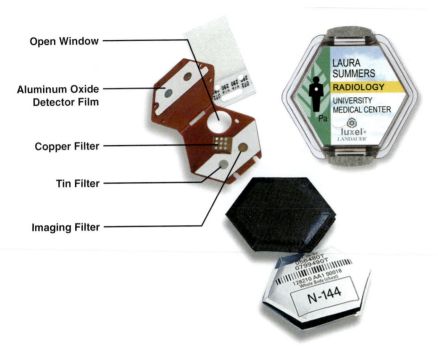

Open Window

Aluminum Oxide Detector Film

Copper Filter

Tin Filter

Imaging Filter

FIGURE 6–8
OSL dosimeter inside view (Courtesy of Landauer, Inc., Glenwood, IL)

using a laser light and becomes luminescent in relation to the amount of radiation it has received (Figure 6–8).

OSLs are capable of measuring different energy ranges. This is determined by the amount of luminescence detected in the areas underneath the filters. These various ranges of energy correspond to deep, eye, and shallow doses.

OSLs are sensitive to approximately 1 mrem. This makes their use especially desirable when monitoring pregnant workers.

Advantages of OSLs:

- Dose measurement range very wide: 1 mrem to 1,000 mrem
- Accuracy +/− 15% for shallow and deep exposures
- Precision within +/− 1.0 mrem
- Energy range 5 keV to over 40 MeV
- Complete re-analysis available – can be restimulated many times
- Bar coding, color coding, graphic formats, and body location icons provide identification
- Bimonthly readout offered
- Tamper-proof sealed badge
- Not affected by heat, moisture, or pressure
- Services include badges for whole body, collar, waist, wrist, and tinge exposure to X-rays, gamma rays, and beta particles
- Reports available in a great variety of forms

Disadvantages of OSLs:

- More expensive than film badges and TLDs

Notes:

Pocket Dosimeters

Pocket dosimeters are a very sensitive type of personnel monitoring device. They provide an instantaneous reading, but must be recalibrated daily. Also, they are capable of only a predetermined range. If exposure exceeds this range, any additional amounts of exposure cannot be documented.

Externally, a pocket dosimeter resembles a fountain pen. It has a pocket clip for attaching to the person's clothing (Figure 6–9). Inside the dosimeter is an **ionization chamber**. The chamber has a positive and a negative electrode. The electrodes and chamber are given a positive charge before use. There is a stationary electrode, and a moving electrode that is referred to as a hair or fiber. Giving a charge to the device with a charging base causes the fiber to be electrostatically repelled from a central electrode. This charge is calibrated until the fiber is set at zero on a visible scale. Ionization of air by radiation causes the hair to move. X- or gamma-radiation ionizes the air within the chamber, which neutralizes the charges present on the fiber and electrode. As the number of negative ions in the chamber increase, the charge on the hair reduces. This causes the hair to move closer to the stationary electrode. Pocket dosimeters are read by viewing a scale through an eyepiece located on the end of the dosimeter.

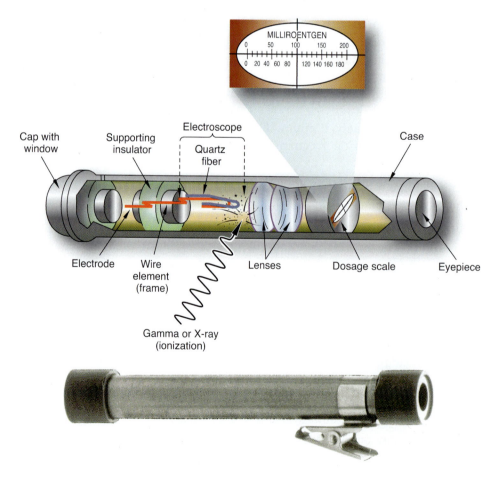

FIGURE 6–9
Pocket dosimeter with cutaway (Courtesy of Bushberg, J. T., Seibert, J. A., Leidholdt, E. M., & Boone, J. M. [1994].
The essential physics of medical imaging. Baltimore: Lippincott Williams & Wilkins.)

Pocket dosimeters are normally used only in emergency situations in which an immediate reading is necessary. They may give false readings if subjected to trauma or high humidity.

Advantages of pocket dosimeters:

- Provides an immediate exposure reading
- Sensitive to exposures up to 200 mR
- Can be reset to record individual exposure readings

Disadvantages of pocket dosimeters:

- Does not provide a permanent legal record of exposure
- Bumping or shock to unit can cause false high readings

Dosimetry Report

Film badges, TLDs, and OSLs are normally collected on a monthly basis, and personnel are supplied with new monitors. The used monitors are sent to the supplier for processing and exposure calculations.

Approximately one month after monitors have been returned to the supplier, the RSO receives a dosimetry report (Figure 6–10).

Notes:

SAMPLE ORGANIZATION
RADIATION SAFETY OFFICER
1000 HIGH TECH AVENUE
GLENWOOD, IL 60425

LANDAUER®

Landauer, Inc. 2 Science Road Glenwood, Illinois 60425-1586
Telephone: (708) 755-7000 Facsimile: (708) 755-7016
www.landauerinc.com

luxel®

RADIATION DOSIMETRY REPORT

ACCOUNT NO.	SERIES CODE	ANALYTICAL WORK ORDER	REPORT DATE	DOSIMETER RECEIVED	REPORT TIME IN WORK DAYS	PAGE NO.
103702	RAD	9920800151	06/11/04	06/07/04	4	1

PARTICIPANT NUMBER	NAME ID NUMBER / BIRTH DATE	SEX	DOSIMETER	USE	RADIATION QUALITY	DOSE EQUIVALENT (MREM) FOR PERIODS SHOWN BELOW			QUARTERLY ACCUMULATED DOSE EQUIVALENT (MREM)			YEAR TO DATE DOSE EQUIVALENT (MREM)			LIFETIME DOSE EQUIVALENT (MREM)			RECORDS FOR YEAR	INCEPTION DATE (MM/YY)
						DEEP DDE	EYE LDE	SHALLOW SDE	DEEP DDE	EYE LDE	SHALLOW SDE	DEEP DDE	EYE LDE	SHALLOW SDE	DEEP DDE	EYE LDE	SHALLOW SDE		
FOR MONITORING PERIOD:						05/01/04 - 05/31/04			QTR 2			2004							
0000H	CONTROL CONTROL CONTROL		Ja Pa U	CNTRL CNTRL CNTRL		M M	M M	M M M										5	07/97 07/97 07/97
00191	ADDISON, JOHN 336235619 08/31/1968	M	Ja	WHBODY	PN P NF	90 60 30	90 60 30	90 60 30	90 60 30	90 60 30	90 60 30	100 70 30	100 70 30	100 70 30	200 170 30	200 170 30	200 170 30	5	07/97
00192	JORGENSON, MIKE 471740095 10/04/1968	M	Pa U	WHBODY RFINGR		M	M	M M	M	M	M M	M	M	M 70	M	M	M 100	5	07/97 07/97
00193	THOMAS, LEE 384846378 11/22/1964	M	Pa U	WHBODY RFINGR		ABSENT ABSENT			M	M	M M	M	M	M M	M	M	M M	5	07/97 07/97
00196	WALKER, JANE 587336640 06/09/1960	F	Pa	WHBODY		3	3	3	12	11	11	12	11	11	22	21	21	5	11/97
00197	EDWARD, CHRIS 489635774 02/14/1966	M	Pa	WHBODY		M	M	M	M	M	M	M	M	M	M	M	M	5	01/98
00198	ZERR, ROBERT 982446591 07/15/1945	M	Pa	WHBODY NOTE		40 CALCULATED	40	40	160	160	160	200	200	200	240	240	240	5	07/98
00199	ADAMS, JANE 335148621 08/25/1951	F	Pa	WHBODY		M	M	M	M	M	M	9	10	12	9	10	12	5	07/98
00200	MEYER, STEVE 416395887 03/21/1947	M	Pa Pa U	COLLAR WAIST ASSIGN NOTE RFINGR	PL	105 M 4 ASSIGNED DOSE BASED ON EDE 1 CALCULATION	105 M 105	105 M 105 140	6	162	165 400	11	327	334 690	51	1247	1284 2180	5	08/98 08/98 08/98
00202	HARRIS, KATHY 352235619 06/15/1972	F	Pa U	WHBODY RFINGR		M	M	M M	M	M	M M	M	M	M 30	M	M	M 30	4	02/99 02/99

QUALITY CONTROL RELEASE: VS 20 - PR 6774 - RPT130 - N1 - 02013

M: MINIMAL REPORTING SERVICE OF 1 MREM
ELECTRONIC MEDIA TO FOLLOW THIS REPORT

NVLAP®
NVLAP LAB CODE 100518-0**

FIGURE 6–10
Dosimetery report (Courtesy of Landauer, Inc., Glenwood, IL)

These reports are posted in an area where they can be reviewed by personnel for review of their occupational exposures.

The following information is contained on the dosimetry report:

- personnel ID number
- monitor type (film badge, TLD, or OSL)
- employee name and social security number
- birth date and sex
- exposure period
- radiation quality (for example, X-rays, beta particles, neutron)
- current exposure
- cumulative quarterly exposure
- cumulative annual exposure
- cumulative total exposure
- unused part of permissible accumulated dose

Dosimetry exposure figures are listed in millirems. An M on the dosimetry report means a minimal or possibly no exposure.

Should a monitored employee change employment, his employer must transfer the cumulative total exposures and the unused part of the permissible accumulated dose for this person to his new employer.

If the RSO determines that an employee has received an overexposure based on the dosimetry report, the employee must be counseled by the RSO, and documentation placed in the employee's personnel file in case of the need for any future reference. The institution's radiation safety program should have a definition of the nature of an overexposure, as determined by the RSO. Guidelines for the facility's monitoring program are also established by the RSO. Any questions that arise about an institution's radiation safety program should be directed to the RSO. An RSO may be a medical physicist, health physicist, radiologist, or other person qualified through adequate training and experience. The RSO's duties include:

- receiving, using, and disposal of radioactive material;
- conducting radiation surveys;
- monitoring personnel and areas;
- testing for leaking radiation;
- designing protective shielding;
- responding to radiation-related emergencies; and
- radioactive spill decontamination.

Radiation Survey Instruments

Radiation survey instruments are used to detect and measure radiation. Commonly used instruments include the Geiger-Muller detector and the ionization chamber-type survey meter (cutie pie).

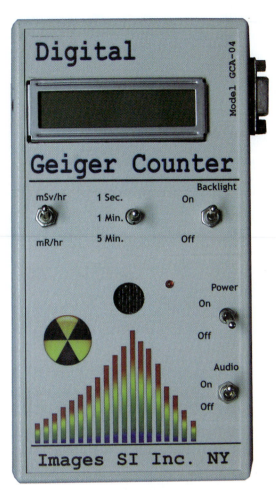

FIGURE 6–11
Geiger-Muller counter (Courtesy of Images Scientific Instruments, Inc.)

The Geiger-Muller detector, better known as a Geiger counter, is normally used to detect alpha and beta radiation (Figure 6–11). The sensor is a Geiger-Muller tube, an inert gas-filled (usually helium, neon, or argon with halogens added) tube that briefly conducts electricity when a particle or photon of radiation temporarily makes the gas conductive. The tube amplifies this conduction by a cascade effect and puts out a current pulse, which is then often displayed by a needle or lamp and/or audible clicks.

The ionization chamber-type survey meter (cutie pie) measures exposure rate for X-ray, gamma, alpha, and beta radiation (Figure 6–12). This meter, developed in the early 1940s, was given its name due to its tiny size. Based on stable and essentially drift-free electrometer technology, this sensitive ion chamber instrument has high sensitivity for alpha and low-to-high energy beta particles, and to gamma and X-ray radiation. The compact and lightweight instrument is useful for measuring exposure and dose rates, determining shielding effectiveness, checking source containers, monitoring radiation areas, and checking results following decontamination procedures.

Notes:

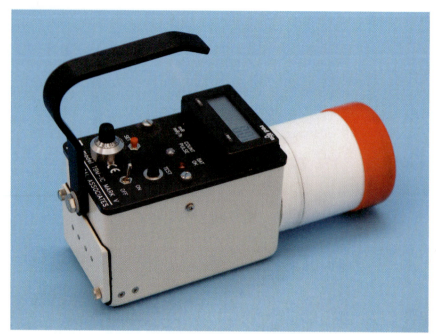

FIGURE 6–12
Cutie pie survey meter (Courtesy of Biodex Medical Systems, Inc.)

DOSE-LIMITING RECOMMENDATIONS

Shortly after the discovery of X-rays by Roentgen in 1895, people came to appreciate the contributions that X-rays would make in medicine. However, it was also soon demonstrated that there would be risks involved. The first fluoroscope users displayed elevated occurrences of skin cancer, cataracts, and lesions of the hands and fingers. In order to keep the health risks to a minimum, standards needed to be instituted.

In the early days of radiology, only short-term effects were acknowledged. Believing that there was a tolerance dose below which there would be no effects, the rationale was that doses should be restricted only in regards to the short term. The 1930s and 1940s saw standards for imaging being established. During this time period, an exposure of one roentgen per day was permissible. Compared with today's exposure levels, this is approximately two times the amount a radiographer would normally acquire in one year.

With the possibility of long-term radiation risks being acknowledged, radiation protection policies are aimed at reducing the likelihood of short- and long-term effects. Present-day radiation protection guidelines are established on the philosophy of keeping exposures **as low as reasonably achievable** (**ALARA**).

Various organizations are involved with radiation protection standards. Their contributions include scientific research reports on radiation and its effects, recommending standards, and making and enforcing guidelines at the state and federal levels. These organizations are identified in Table 6–1. Based on recommendations made by these agencies, radiation exposure limits can be initiated by an act of Congress. Through the Agreement State Program, 34 states have signed formal agreements

TABLE 6-1

Radiation Protection Organizations

Organization	Date Established
International Labour Organization (ILO)	1919
International Commission on Radiological Units and Measurements (ICRU)	1925
International Commission on Radiological Protection (ICRP)	1928
National Council on Radiation Protection and Measurement (NCRP)	1929
United Nations Scientific Committee on Effects of Atomic Radiation (UNSCEAR)	1955
National Research Council Committee on the Biological Effects of Ionizing Radiation (BEIR)	1955
International Atomic Energy Agency (IAEA)	1957
Conference of Radiation Control Program Directors (CRCPD)	1968
U.S. Nuclear Regulatory Commission (NRC), originally established as the U.S. Atomic Energy Commission (AEC)	1940
U.S. Food and Drug Administration (FDA)	1968
U.S. Environmental Protection Agency (EPA)	1970
U.S. Occupational Safety and Health Administration (OSHA)	1971

with the Nuclear Regulatory Commission (NRC) in taking the responsibility to enforce radiation protection guidelines through each state's respective department of health. These 34 states are known as **agreement states**. In non-agreement states, both the NRC and the state are responsible for enforcing radiation protection regulations.

All states, whether they are agreement or non-agreement states, have guidelines for the use of ionizing radiation equipment. Most states act according to regulations designed after the Suggested State Regulations for the Control of Radiation (SSRCR). These recommended regulations are made by the Conference of Radiation Control Program Directors (CRCPD), U.S. Nuclear Regulatory Commission (NRC), U.S. Environmental Protection Agency (EPA), Department of Health and Human Services Public Health Service, and the U.S. Food and Drug Administration (FDA).

Federal government regulations allow diagnostic radiology personnel to receive an annual **effective dose limit** of 5 rem (50 mSv) for whole-body occupational exposure. The public has an annual effective dose limit of 0.5 rem (5 mSv). This amount is 1/10th the amount allowed for people exposed occupationally.

The reason for radiation workers being allowed a larger dose limit is that the radiology workforce is a very small group when compared with the whole population. Hence, radiation workers may receive larger amounts of radiation than the general public acquires. Even though radiation workers may receive more radiation than the general public, the dose equivalent must be kept to a minimum whenever possible.

The effective dose limit for a radiographer during any 13-week period is 3 rem (30 mSv). The annual effective dose limit for the lens of the eye is 15 rem (150 mSv), and for all other organs is 50 rem (500 mSv).

Student radiographers under 18 years of age have an annual effective dose limit of 0.1 rem (1 mSv).

The dose-limiting recommendations during pregnancy are: total effective dose limit = 0.5 rem (5 mSv); effective dose limit for one month = 0.05 rem (0.5 mSv). If the mother received 500 mrem, the embryo or fetus would receive an equivalent of less than 10 mrem.

So that regulatory agencies may dismiss a level of individual risk as negligible risk, an annual **negligible individual dose (NID)** of 1 mrem/yr (0.01 mSv/yr) has been set. Below this effective dose level, reduction of individual exposure is not required.

Table 6–2 summarizes the dose limitations. These values are based on NCRP Report No. 116.

A pregnant employee may choose to voluntarily disclose her pregnancy to the employer, and provide the approximate conception date. This written notification allows her RSO to counsel the employee to follow proper radiation protection guidelines. A pregnant employee by no means should be removed from her duties. The employee's previous exposure history should be reviewed, her work

TABLE 6–2

Annual Dose Limits

Occupational Exposures	Dose Limits
Whole-body	5 rem (50 mSv)
Lens of eye	15 rem (150 mSv)
Skin/extremities	50 rem (500 mSv)
Whole-body cumulative (lifetime)	Age × 1 rem (Age × 10 mSv)
Fetus (nine-month)	0.5 rem (5 mSv)
Fetus (one-month)	0.05 rem (0.5 mSv)
Student < 18 years of age	0.1 rem (1 mSv)
Public Exposure	
Infrequent exposure	0.5 rem (5 mSv)
Frequent exposure	0.1 rem (1 mSv)

environment analyzed to estimate the possibility of receiving exposures that would be greater than the 0.5 rem limit, and finally her work routines altered to lessen the likelihood of risks.

The cumulative whole-body effective dose limit is calculated by multiplying one's age in years by 1 rem (10 mSv).

> **EXAMPLE**
>
> A radiation worker who is age 30 would be allowed a cumulative whole body dose limit of 30 rems. Age (30) × 1 rem = 30 rems.

These occupational exposures are made in keeping with the ALARA principle, that is, maintain radiation exposures as low as reasonably achievable. ALARA suggests that the absolute absorbed dose limit values are to be kept below the maximum amounts allowed. The most effective way for radiographers to do this is to use correct radiation protection procedures, which should include a combination of time, distance, and shielding. Also, the radiographer should utilize accurate centering and collimation of the X-ray beam.

Radiographers should familiarize themselves with approximated doses of representative radiologic exams, as patients may inquire about how much exposure they are receiving. A radiologist may be consulted to converse with the patient about the doses they are receiving.

Table 6–3 lists the representative quantities for various X-ray exams:

The radiographer should know his or her department's protocol regarding the release of such information to patients. It may be that only the radiologist or RSO may release this information.

Patients may not necessarily want to know specifics on exposure, but instead may only want to be assured that the person performing their exam is knowledgeable regarding representative exposures for radiologic exams.

TABLE 6–3

Exposure Quantities for Specific X-ray Exams

Exam	Skin Dose (mrad)	Mean Marrow Dose (mrad)	Gonad Dose (mrad)
PA Chest	10–20	2	<1
AP Abdomen	250–500	30	125
Skull	100–200	10	<1
Extremity	10–200	2	<1
Cervical Spine	150	10	<1
Lumbar Spine	300	60	225
Pelvis	150	20	150

Notes:

Notes:

All facilities that receive accreditation by the **Joint Commission** are required to monitor doses from diagnostic radiologic exams. It is also recommended by the Center for Devices and Radiological Health (CDRH) that diagnostic radiologic institutions be familiar with the amounts of radiation that are received by patients. Patient doses are usually reported in one of three methods: skin dose, gonadal dose, and bone marrow dose. **Skin dose**, also referred to as **entrance skin exposure (ESE)**, is a measure of the radiation to a patient's skin at the entrance surface. Skin dose is the type of method most often used, because it is easy to measure. To get a skin dose measurement, a TLD is placed on the patient's skin in the center of the primary X-ray beam. Because of suspected genetic response to ionizing radiation, **gonadal dose** is vital. Measuring the dose to the gonads is also easy to measure. **Bone marrow dose** is critical as bone marrow is thought to be the target organ responsible for radiation-induced leukemia.

Patient doses can be determined by utilizing the known output intensity from the X-ray tube. The output intensity of an X-ray tube varies directly with the mAs (milliampere second), directly with the square of the kVp (kilovolt peak), and inversely with the square of the distance from the focal spot.

$$\text{Output intensity} = \frac{K(mAs)kVp^2}{D^2}$$

The measurement of K, which is a constant, is recorded at 70 kVp and 40 inches. Once K is determined,

$$\text{Output intensity (mR)} = K(mR/mAs)(mAs_2)\frac{(kVp_2)}{(70)^2}\frac{(40 \text{ inches})^2}{(d_2)^2}$$

K = recorded value at 70 kVp and 40 inches

mAs_2 = new technique

kVp_2 = new technique

d_2 = new SID (source-image receptor distance)

EXAMPLE

The determined value for K is 10 mR/mAs at 70 kVp and 40 inches SID. For an extremity, 3 mAs and 55 kVp are used. What is the intensity?

$$(10 \text{ mR/mAs})(3 \text{ mAs})\frac{(55)^2}{(70)^2}\frac{(40)^2}{(40)^2} = 10 \text{ mR} \times 3 \times 0.6 \times 1 = 30 \text{ mR}$$

The ESE (entrance skin exposure) for an X-ray projection can be approximated by using an ionization chamber. A digital dosimeter is exposed to the technique used for the specified projection. The formula for calculating an estimated ESE dose is:

$$\frac{\text{dosimeter exposure (mR)}}{\text{ESE (mR)}} = \frac{SSD^2}{SDD^2}$$

SSD = source to skin distance

SDD = source to detector distance

If a radiographer doubles the mAs, the radiation intensity doubles. Doubling the mAs also doubles the ESE (entrance skin exposure), as long as other factors are held constant.

The following is the formula for mAs and intensity:

$$\frac{mAs_1}{mAs_1} = \frac{I_1}{I_1}$$

EXAMPLE

If an original intensity was 200 mR, and the mAs value is increased from 10 to 20 mAs, what happens to the intensity? Doubling mAs should also double intensity.

$$\frac{10}{20} = \frac{200}{x} \qquad 10x = 4,000 \qquad x = 400 \text{ mR}$$

EXAMPLE

If an original intensity was 200 mR, and the mAs value is decreased from 100 mAs to 50 mAs, what happens to intensity? Decreasing mAs should also decrease intensity.

$$\frac{100}{50} = \frac{200}{x} \qquad 100x = 10,000 \qquad x = 100 \text{ mR}$$

Changing kVp affects radiation intensity by the square of the ratios of the kVps. The following is the formula for kVp and radiation intensity:

$$\frac{(kVp_1)^2}{(kVp_2)^2} = \frac{I_1}{I_2}$$

EXAMPLE

If 50 kVp produces an intensity of 200 mR, what will be the intensity at 100 kVp if no other factors are changed? Increasing kVp should also increase intensity.

$$\frac{50^2}{(100)^2} = \frac{200}{x} \qquad \frac{1}{4} = \frac{200}{x} \qquad x = 800 \text{ mR}$$

EXAMPLE

If 100 kVp produces an intensity of 800 mR, what will be the intensity at 70 kVp if no other factors are changed? Decreasing kVp should also decrease intensity.

$$\frac{(100)^2}{(70)^2} = \frac{800}{x} \qquad \frac{100}{49} = \frac{800}{x} \qquad 100x = 39,20 \qquad x = 392 \text{ mR}$$

PRINCIPLES OF PERSONNEL EXPOSURE REDUCTION

Reduction of an individual's exposure to ionizing radiation may be accomplished by application of three basic principles: (1) reduce the amount of time spent in the vicinity of the radiation source while it is operating, (2) increase the distance between the radiation source and the individual to be protected, and (3) interpose a shielding material, which will attenuate the radiation from the source. These three basic principles are sometimes referred to as the three cardinal rules of radiation protection.

Time

X-ray imaging equipment produces radiation only during the actual exposure used to form the image during a procedure. The time of exposure on a per-image basis is very short (typically much less than 1 second) during radiographic procedures. During fluoroscopic procedures, which are used when dynamic information is required, the X-ray source may be on (usually intermittently) for several minutes. To minimize exposure to radiation, individuals should reduce the amount of time they spend in the vicinity of an operable radiation source. The simplest way to do this is to ascertain whether their presence is needed during the procedure. Whenever possible, individuals should remain behind protective barriers.

Distance

Increasing the distance between the individual and the source of radiation is an effective method to reduce exposure to radiation. As distance from the source of radiation is increased, the radiation level will decrease significantly. Maximizing the distance from an operable source of radiation is a particularly effective method of exposure reduction during mobile radiographic and fluoroscopic procedures. Distance utilizes the inverse square law.

Shielding

Shielding is used when neither time nor distance is effective in achieving the desired degree of reduction in exposure. By interposing any material between the source of radiation and the point at which it is desired to reduce the exposure, a certain reduction in exposure will be achieved. The degree of exposure reduction will depend on the physical characteristics of the material (atomic number, density, and thickness). For fixed X-ray imaging facilities the most common materials are lead and concrete. Such facilities are designed in accordance with specific recommendations (NCRP Report No. 49) depending on the configuration of the equipment, its intended use, and the surrounding area. Additional devices, such as mobile shields, lead-equivalent aprons, and lead-equivalent gloves should be used when it is not possible to take advantage of fixed structural barriers.

STRUCTURAL SHIELDING CONSTRUCTION

The two types of fixed barriers are primary and secondary. **Primary protective barriers**, which are located perpendicular to the line of travel of the primary X-ray beam, in radiography up to 140 kVp, should consist of 1/16 inch lead (Pb) or equivalent, which extends up

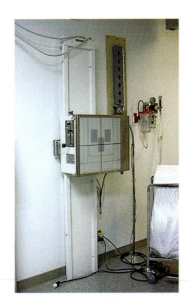

FIGURE 6–13
Primary protective barrier behind wall Bucky

at least 7 feet from the floor when the X-ray tube is 5 to 7 feet from the wall (Figure 6–13).

Secondary protective barriers, which are located parallel to the line of travel of the primary X-ray beam, cover areas exposed only to scattered and leakage radiation, and require 1/32 inch lead (Pb) or equivalent under the same operating conditions stated above. Plaster or concrete often serves as a secondary barrier without added lead.

Control booths are regarded as secondary barriers. X-rays have scattered at least two times before hitting the control booth, which causes a reduction of the X-ray beam to one-millionth of its original value.

The radiographer can observe the patient by looking through the lead glass window in the control booth. This leaded glass observation window should have the same lead equivalency as the adjacent wall. Lead glass is typically four times as thick as sheet lead for equivalent protection. Observation windows may be obtained in lead equivalencies from 0.3 to 2 mm. The average lead glass window of the shielded control booth consists of 1.5 mm Pb equivalent (Figure 6–14).

The exposure cord for the control booth must be short enough so that an exposure can be made only when the radiographer is entirely behind the control booth barrier. Control booth walls must be at least 7 feet high, and should be mounted permanently to the floor. If there is a door that is used as a necessary component of the control booth, it should be electrically interlocked with the control panel so that X-rays cannot be produced without the door being closed.

In addition to the primary and secondary protective barriers previously mentioned, the X-ray tube itself must be enclosed by a lead-lined metal covering, the required shielding being approximately 1.5 mm (1/16 inch) Pb. This **protective tube housing** serves to reduce leakage radiation to an assigned safe level (Figure 6–15). Leakage from the X-ray tube housing should not exceed 100 mR/hr at 3 feet (1 meter).

Notes:

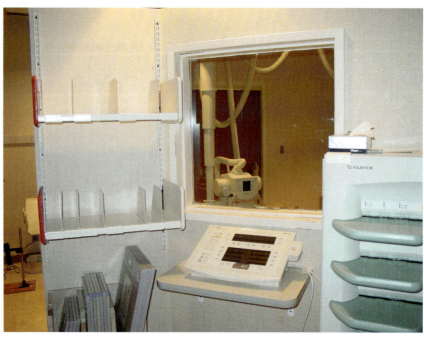

FIGURE 6–14
Lead-lined control booth

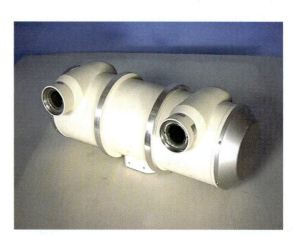

FIGURE 6–15
X-ray tube housing

During radiography and fluoroscopic procedures, at 1 meter from the patient, the beam intensity is reduced by a factor of 1,000, to approximately 0.1% of the original beam intensity.

Factors that determine protective barrier thickness include distance, **time of occupancy (T), workload (W),** and **use (U)**.

Barrier thickness depends on the distance between the radiation source and the barrier. The greater the distance between the radiation source and the barrier, the less lead thickness needed for the barrier.

Time of occupancy factor (T) denotes the amount of time a hospital area is occupied by people. Occupancy factor (T) is divided into two types: controlled and uncontrolled. A **controlled area** is an area occupied by radiation personnel. This area is always given an occupancy factor of 1. This is an implication that a radiation worker is always present.

An **uncontrolled area** is one that is occupied by non-radiation personnel, that is, the general public. These areas are designated as either full, partial, or occasional, depending on their purpose. Stairways, unattended elevators, and outside areas are examples of uncontrolled areas.

The uncontrolled area occupancy factor value depends on the use of the area, for example, hallways = (T) factor of 1/4, stairways and unattended elevators = (T) factor of 1/16.

Controlled area design limits require barriers to reduce the exposure rate to less than 100 mrem/week. Uncontrolled area design limits require barriers to reduce the exposure rate to less than 10 mrem/week. Thus, uncontrolled walls must have approximately a tenth-value layer of lead as compared to that of a controlled wall.

Barrier thickness depends on the radiation level activity in that room. The more exams performed, the thicker the barrier needed. This characteristic, called workload (W), which takes into account weekly average tube current and tube operating time, is measured in milliampere-minutes/week (mA-min/wk). A small office may have workloads of less than 100 mA-min/wk, whereas a busy hospital may have a general-purpose X-ray room with workloads as high as 500 mA-min/wk.

EXAMPLE

Plans for a private radiologist office call for two X-ray rooms. Patient load for each room is estimated to be 10 patients/day, with each patient averaging 4 films taken at 70 kVp, 70 mAs. What will be the projected workload of each room?

10 patients/day × 5 days/week = 50 patients/week

50 patients/wk × 4 films/patient = 200 films/week

200 films/week × 70 mAs/film = 14,000 mAs/week

$$14,000 \text{ mAs/week} \times \frac{1 \text{ minute}}{60 \text{ seconds}} = 233.3 \text{ mA-min/week}$$

The use factor (U) is the percentage of time that the X-ray beam is energized and directed toward a particular wall. The NCRP recommends that primary wall barriers be given a use factor of 1, and that primary floor barriers be given a use factor of 1. A wall that is not a primary barrier would be given a use factor of 1/4. Because scattered and leakage radiation are present 100% of the time when the X-ray tube is energized, the use factor for secondary barriers is assigned a factor of 1.

USE OF PROTECTIVE GARMENTS

Because lead's high atomic number ensures that most scattered photons are absorbed, it is the material most often chosen for shielding.

Shields are evaluated by half-value layers (HVLs). HVLs refer to the lead thicknesses that will reduce the intensity of radiation to 50%.

Lead aprons should be worn by all radiographers performing mobile and/or fluoroscopic procedures, and if holding a patient during an exposure (Figure 6–16). Aprons are composed of lead-impregnated vinyl or rubber. Lead aprons are manufactured in thicknesses of 0.25, 0.5, and 1 mm lead equivalencies. X-ray attenuation at 75 kVp for a 1 mm Pb equivalent apron is 99% (Figure 6–17).

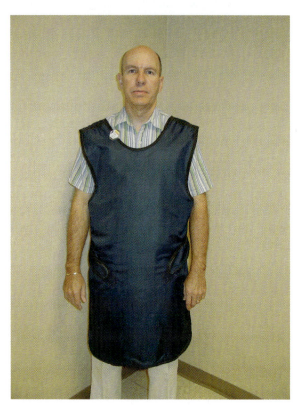

FIGURE 6–16
Lead apron

Lead Apron Effectiveness

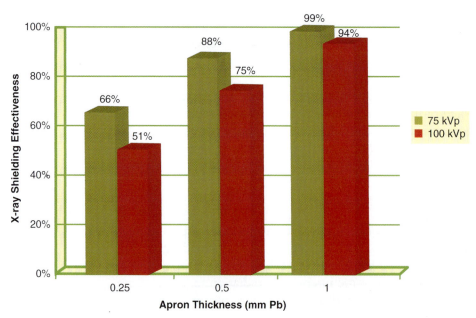

FIGURE 6–17
Lead apron effectiveness

Presuming the person wearing a lead apron is facing the primary X-ray beam, approximately 3/4 of the body's active bone marrow is covered. There are full wrap-around aprons available for personnel who are not always able to be facing the primary beam.

The greater the lead equivalency of an apron, the heavier it is for the person wearing it, which could possibly lead to back problems. Aprons with a 1-mm lead equivalency may weigh up to 25 pounds.

To offset the weight factor of lead-impregnated aprons, manufacturers have begun to make aprons of composite materials. The aprons are made of a combination of barium, tungsten, and lead. This combination of materials maintains comparable radiation attenuation with lead aprons, and also is reduced in weight by almost 30%.

When wearing a lead apron, the personnel monitor should be worn at the collar level on the outside of the apron.

Maternity aprons are available for pregnant personnel (Figure 6–18). These aprons maintain 0.5 mm Pb equivalent protection throughout, and also contain an extra band of lead that covers the patient the entire width of the apron from the xiphoid process to slightly below the symphysis pubis. The additional band of lead provides the fetus with 1 mm Pb equivalent protection.

Notes:

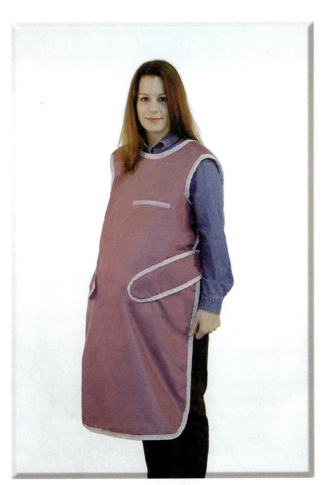

FIGURE 6–18
Maternity apron (Courtesy of Pacific Northwest X-Ray, Inc.)

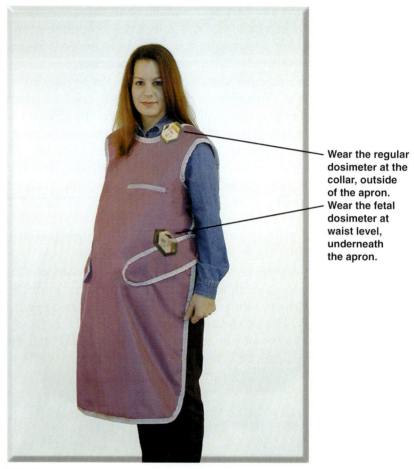

Wear the regular dosimeter at the collar, outside of the apron.

Wear the fetal dosimeter at waist level, underneath the apron.

FIGURE 6–19
Double-badging pregnant employee (Courtesy of Pacific Northwest X-Ray, Inc.)

Pregnant radiographers should be provided with two personnel monitors (Figure 6–19). When wearing a lead apron, one should be worn at the collar level on the outside of the apron, and the other should be worn at the waist level on the inside of the apron.

If it is necessary for personnel to have their hands in the beam, lead gloves with a minimum lead equivalency of 0.25 mm must be worn (Figure 6–20). Sterile gloves that are radiation resistant are also manufactured. These are composed of lead-lined rubber. The thinness of the sterile glove permits more flexibility than is available with ordinary lead gloves, but they do not have the attenuation that regular lead gloves do.

Radiologists receive high radiation doses to the thyroid when performing fluoroscopy. Thyroid shields of 0.5 mm lead equivalency are available to protect the thyroid area of personnel. Wearing a thyroid shield during fluoroscopy reduces the dose to the individual by a factor of 10 (Figure 6–21).

Although protective eyewear has been recommended to be worn by radiologists during fluoroscopy to protect the eyes from cataractogenic effects of radiation, this need has never been established.

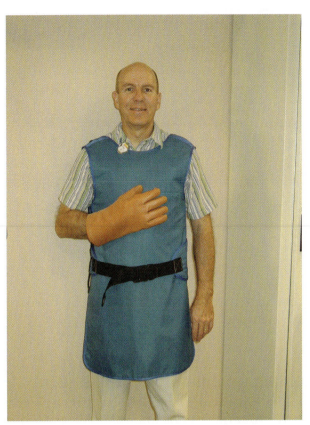

FIGURE 6–20
Lead gloves

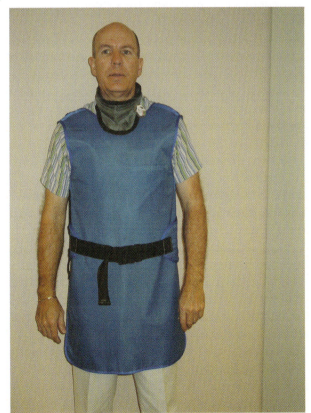

FIGURE 6–21
Thyroid shield

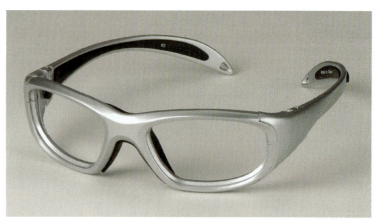

FIGURE 6–22
Lead glasses (Courtesy of Pacific Northwest X-Ray, Inc.)

Protective eyeglasses are available with lead equivalency protection of 0.35 mm (Figure 6–22).

MOBILE EXAM CONSIDERATIONS

It is crucial that the radiographer initiate effective communication with the patient during a mobile radiographic exam. Just as when performing an exam in the department, the radiographer should appraise the patient's condition and his or her ability to cooperate.

Before the radiographer makes an exposure during mobile radiography, they should instruct any people who are not required to be in the room during the exposure to leave the area. Anyone who is not able to leave the area during the exposure, including patients, must be provided with protective shielding. After the exposure is done, the radiographer should instruct anyone who was asked to leave the area that the exposure has been completed and that the room may be re-entered.

In order to receive the least amount of **scattered radiation** during a mobile exam, the radiographer should position himself or herself at right angles to the scattering object (patient). Taking into consideration the radiation protection factors of distance and shielding, this is where the radiographer will receive the least amount of scattered radiation. The radiographer is also advised to take a position around a corner during the exposure. When doing so, any radiation that does reach the radiographer will have scattered at least two times. For each scattering effect, the radiation exposure is reduced by a factor of 0.01%. The radiographer would receive the greatest amount of radiation by standing beside the X-ray machine, because of backscatter exiting the patient.

Lead aprons should be worn at all times by radiographers performing mobile radiographic procedures. These lead aprons must have a minimum lead thickness equivalency of 0.5 mm. If the radiographers' hands have to be placed in the primary beam, lead gloves must be worn. These gloves must have a minimum lead thickness equivalency of 0.25 mm.

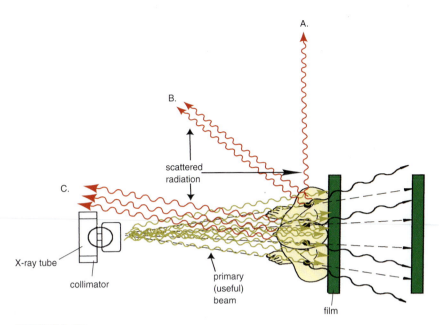

FIGURE 6–23
Source of radiation during mobile exam

   The mobile unit exposure switch must permit the radiographer to obtain a distance of at least 6 feet from the X-ray tube, patient, and **useful beam**. Utilizing distance takes advantage of the inverse square law. It is recommended that the radiographer stand at least 6 feet from the X-ray source. Sources of potential radiation during an exposure include both the X-ray tube and the patient (Figure 6–23).

   During mobile procedures, the radiographer should use a combination of the three cardinal principles of radiation protection: time, distance, and shielding.

- Reduce time: While the X-ray tube is operating, keep the amount of time spent in the area of the tube to a minimum.
- Increase distance: Keep as large a distance as possible between the energized X-ray tube and the exposed patient.
- Utilize shielding: Place lead shielding between the energized X-ray tube and the exposed person.

   Table 6–4 summarizes some rules to remember when using mobile radiography.

FLUOROSCOPIC EXAM CONSIDERATIONS

A lead apron of at least 0.5 mm Pb equivalent must worn by all persons (other than the patient) who are present in the fluoroscopic room during exposure. (See Figure 6–16.) An apron designed to cover the front and sides of the body is usually sufficient, although a wrap-around apron for both front and back should be considered if the radiographer is required to turn his or her back to the patient and X-ray tube during the procedure. Radiographers assisting during fluoroscopy must develop the ability to always keep the front of their body with the lead apron facing the patient and tube. If the hands

Notes:

TABLE 6–4

Radiation Protection Rules for Mobile Radiography

1. Recognize a duty to protect your patient, health professionals, physicians, the public, and yourself.
2. Request the public, health professionals, physicians, and other patients to leave the immediate area prior to exposure.

    (Always inform these persons that you will be finished in a moment, request them to remain nearby, and inform them promptly when you are finished.)

3. Announce in a loud voice your intent to make each exposure and permit sufficient time for others to leave.
4. Carry at least two lead aprons: one for yourself, the other for your patient. Any assistants must have an apron as well.
5. Never place your hand or any other body part within the primary beam.
6. Provide gonadal protection for your patient.
7. Achieve maximum distance from the patient (not the tube) immediately prior to exposure, in accordance with rules requiring the use of a 6-foot cord on mobile units.
8. Label and handle each cassette carefully to avoid repeats.

(From Carlton, R. & Adler, A. [2006]. *Principles of Radiographic Imaging: An Art and a Science* [4th ed.]. Albany, NY: Thomson Delmar Learning.)

must be placed within the primary beam, lead gloves of at least 0.25 mm Pb equivalent must be worn. (See Figure 6–20.)

The primary source of exposure to the radiographer and radiologist is the patient. It is worth noting that the highest energy scatter occurs at a 90° angle to the incident beam and that the patient on an X-ray table is usually at the same level (90° from a primary photon angle of incidence) as the gonads of the radiographer. It is also worth remembering that according to the inverse square law, a single step back from the patient will decrease the dose exponentially (Figure 6–24). The slot immediately under the tabletop where the Bucky tray is positioned for diagnostic radiography is also at the gonadal level. Fluoroscopic units must have a lead shield to cover this slot. This lead shield is termed the Bucky slot cover, which is brought into position by moving the Bucky tray to the head or foot of the table prior to beginning fluoroscopy (Figure 6–25). Strips of lead rubber that form a drape are positioned between the fluoroscopist and patient to absorb the majority of the patient scatter (Figure 6–26). The radiographer has one advantage during fluoroscopy in that he or she may position himself or herself behind the radiologist. This not only adds an additional lead apron, but the entire body of the fluoroscopist is there to protect the radiographer.

Fluoroscopy units with cassette spot filming devices are available in front- and rear-loading models. The front-loading models require the fluoroscopist to eject the cassette and lift the arm to permit the radiographer to remove the exposed cassette and insert an unexposed

Due to
not be
loading

Th
by usii
fluoros
Only v
fluoros

Th
(30 cm
(38 cm

Th
2.5 mn

Th
barrier

A o
an aud
used. T
each n

Th
10 R/n
fluoros
mode,

Th
fluoro
of inte
patient

Th
fluoros
roscop
whene
The u:
person

FIGURE 6–29
Benefit of increasing

EXAMPLE

If the radiograph
6 feet from the s
a factor of 4, ac

Of the thi
inverse square
radiographer fi

PATIENT IM

Immobilizatioi
motion. Involu
time with a hig

A combina
tioning aids sh
sandbags, and
bands, and tap

Immobiliz
cooperate. Th
patient's abilit
then decided
should be exp

As a last r
Radiographer
tion. No one

INVEI

By inc
radiog
exposu
This la
a poin
of the

Th

wh

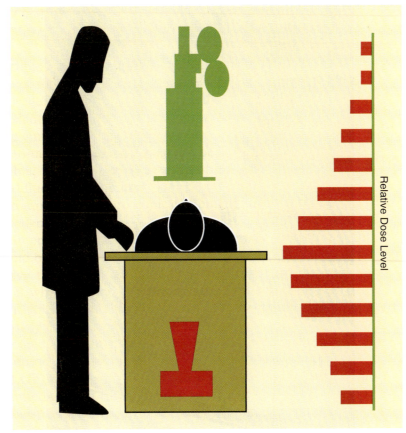

FIGURE 6–24
Scatter radiation profile

Relative Dose Level

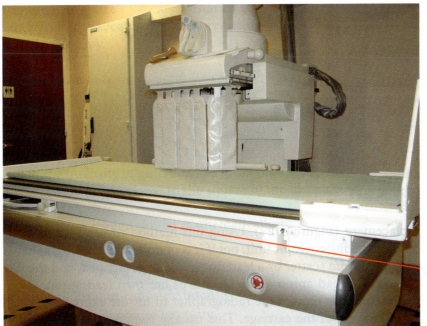

FIGURE 6–25
Bucky slot cover

Notes:

Note   Notes: ————   Notes: ————————

The first choice for holding a patient is a friend or relative, preferably a male, since a male cannot be pregnant. Nonradiology hospital employees are the next choice. The final choice for holding patients would be radiology personnel.

Persons holding a patient for an exposure must be furnished with a lead apron and lead gloves. The person holding the patient should be instructed to not stand in the useful/primary beam during the exposure. It is recommended by the ICRP that the person holding the patient be above the reproductive age. Under no circumstances should a pregnant female be used to support or hold a patient during an exposure.

Many medical facilities keep a daily logbook that contains the patient's name, the date the exam was performed, exposure technique factors, number of images taken, and radiographer's initials. Also recorded is the name of human immobilizer used, and during which exposures they were utilized.

If physical restraint is to be used on a patient, you must first get their consent. Failing to do so may result in legal consequences.

Permitting patients to cooperate if they are able to do so is recommended. Achieving patient cooperation and consent may save you from having to do repeat images. All radiographers should employ this professional approach when giving patient instructions.

KEY CONCEPTS

- Radiation protection is used to limit the amount of radiation an individual is exposed to, thus warding off ill effects of the radiation exposure.

- Personnel monitors are devices worn by radiographers to measure the amount of radiation they are exposed to on a daily basis. Personnel monitor reports summarize the amount of radiation an individual is exposed to in a specific period. The radiation safety officer is responsible for maintaining the protection of personnel, monitoring personnel exposures, testing for radiation leaks, developing shielding apparatus, responding to emergencies involving radiation exposure, and coordinating the decontamination of radiation spills.

- Dose-limiting recommendations were developed to ensure that personnel are exposed to only the minimum levels to maintain health. This is calculated by multiplying one's age in years by 1 rem.

- Structural shielding construction creates areas that provide the maximum amount of safety for the radiographer by limiting the exposure of radiation by use of barriers. Factors to consider when developing these areas are distance, time of occupancy, workload, and use.

- To reduce the amount of exposure of the radiographer during a mobile exam, the radiographer should wear a lead

---

American Society of Radiologic Technologists

CURRICULUM

The material presented in this chapter reflects the following area(s) of the ASRT Curriculum Guide:

Topic:

Radiation Protection

Content:

I. Introduction

II. Units, Detection, and Measurement

III. Surveys, Regulatory/Advisory Agencies, and Regulations

IV. Personnel Monitoring

V. Application

apron, be at least 6 feet away from the patient, and position himself at right angles to the patient. It is also advisable to take a position around a corner from the patient.

- To minimize exposure of the radiographer during a fluoroscopic exam, the radiographer should try to increase the distance from the table.
- Increasing one's distance decreases exposure as a result of the radiation scattering.
- The inverse square law is used to measure the decrease in exposure by increasing distance. The intensity of radiation at a given distance is inversely proportional to the square of the distance of the object from the source.
- Lead aprons, lead gloves, thyroid shields, and protective eyewear should be worn to protect against exposure to radiation.
- When a patient needs to be immobilized, individuals who are not regularly exposed to radiation should be used first. Radiographic personnel should be used only as a last resort. Positioning aids can also be used such as tape, sponges, sandbags, and foam pads.

Notes:

REVIEW QUESTIONS & EXERCISES

Crossword Puzzle

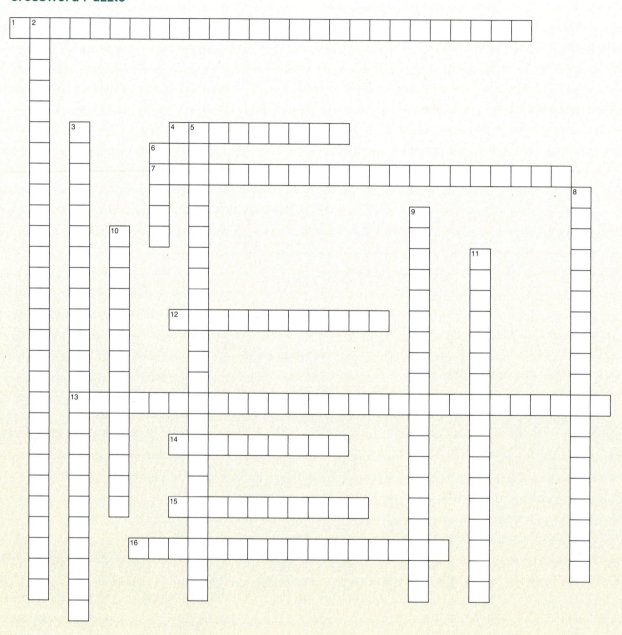

Across

1. A fixed barrier that is located parallel to the line of travel of the primary X-ray beam.

4. A type of dosimeter consisting of radiation dosimetry film to determine the amount of exposure personnel have received.

7. The response of human cells exposed to radiation within minutes, days, or weeks of exposure.

12. Exposure control switch that is either a foot pedal or a hand switch.

13. A device containing lithium fluoride or calcium fluoride crystals to calculate the amount of personnel exposure.

14. Measurement of ionizing radiation doses to personnel.

15. The primary X-ray beam.

16. An area occupied by non-radiation personnel.

Down

2. The lowest dose of radiation that will maintain health with no ill effects.

3. A fixed barrier that is located perpendicular to the line of travel of the primary X-ray beam.

5. The procedure of periodically activating the fluoroscopic tube.

6. As low as reasonably achievable.

8. Methods used to limit exposure to radiation.

9. Devices used to measure radiation doses.

10. An area occupied by radiation personnel.

11. A tube containing charged positive and negative electrodes. One electrode is stationary, the other is moving. Exposure to ionization is determined by measurement of the moving electrode's movement.

Matching

Match the definition in the right column with the correct term from the left column.

_____ 1. Agreement states

_____ 2. Bone marrow dose

_____ 3. Cumulative timing device

_____ 4. Dose

_____ 5. Early effect of radiation

_____ 6. Entrance skin exposure (ESE)

_____ 7. Gonadal dose

_____ 8. Inverse square law

_____ 9. Joint Commission on the Accreditation of Healthcare Organizations (JCAHO)

_____ 10. Lead equivalent

_____ 11. Pocket dosimeter

_____ 12. Protective tube housing

_____ 13. Scattered radiation

_____ 14. Skin dose

_____ 15. Time of occupancy (T)

_____ 16. Use (U)

_____ 17. Workload (W)

a. The amount of activity of the X-ray machinery

b. Radiation that is dissipated away from the point of origin

c. The amount of time a hospital area is occupied by people

d. The amount of material that is needed to meet the same requirements as a lead barrier

e. The intensity of radiation as a given distance is inversely proportional to the square of the distance of the object from the source

f. A measure of the radiation to the patient at the site of the patient's gonads

g. A measure of the radiation to the patient's skin at the skin entrance surface

h. A device that presets the on time for the tube to only 5-minute increments

i. A measure of the radiation that has been absorbed into the patient's bone marrow

j. Those states that have agreements with the Nuclear Regulatory Commission to take responsibility to enforce radiation protection guidelines through the states' department of health

k. The response of human cells exposed to radiation within minutes, days, or weeks of exposure

l. The lead-lined metal covering of the X-ray beam that serves to reduce leakage radiation

m. Amount of radiation exposure

n. Device that uses an ionization chamber to determine the level of exposure

o. The percentage of time in which the X-ray beam is energized and directed toward a particular wall

p. A measure of the radiation at the skin entrance surface

q. The accrediting body for radiographic facilities

Multiple Choice

1. Guidelines for an institution's radiation monitoring program are established by:
   - a. hospital administrator
   - b. radiation safety officer
   - c. radiology manager
   - d. radiologist

2. Diagnostic radiology personnel may receive an annual dose equivalent of:
   - a. 0.5 rem (5 mSv)
   - b. 1 rem (10 mSv)
   - c. 5 rem (50 mSv0)
   - d. 10 rem (150 mSv)

3. The exposure cord on a mobile unit must be at least _____ in length.
   - a. 1 foot
   - b. 3 feet
   - c. 6 feet
   - d. 10 feet

4. A Bucky slot cover should be at least how thick?
   - a. 0.025 mm Pb equivalent
   - b. 0.25 mm Pb equivalent
   - c. 0.025 mm Al equivalent
   - d. 0.25 mm Al equivalent

5. Protective lead gloves must have a minimum lead equivalency of at least _____ lead.
   - a. 0.025 mm
   - b. 0.25 mm
   - c. 0.5 mm
   - d. 1.0 mm

6. Which of the following people should be used to hold a patient who needs physical support during the exposure?
   - a. radiographer
   - b. friend
   - c. pregnant person
   - d. nurse

7. Primary protective barriers must consist of _____ inch lead.
   - a. 1/16
   - b. 1/8
   - c. ¼
   - d. 1/32

SITUATIONAL JUDGMENT TESTING

A physician has ordered an upright PA and lateral chest series on an elderly patient who cannot stand. Who would you choose to hold this patient in the upright position?
   - a. nurse
   - b. pregnant family member
   - c. adult male family member
   - d. radiographer

EXPLORING THE WEB

1. Search the Web for regulations regarding occupational exposure to radiation. What agencies regulate occupational exposure? Is your state an agreement state? Does your state enforce any regulations that differ from the national standard?

_____

_____

_____

_____

2. Search the Web for additional information on safety in the workplace for radiographers. What did you find? Did you discover any additional tips on maintaining a safe work environment?

_____

_____

_____

_____

3. Search the Web for dosimetry. Explain how this works. Go to the Web sites of companies that manufacture dosimeters. What products are available for the protection of the radiographer? What are the pros and cons of the products available?

_____

_____

_____

_____

CASE STUDY

You are about to perform a mobile X-ray exam on your patient. Discuss how you should utilize the three cardinal principles of radiation protection for you and your patient.

_____

_____

_____

_____

_____

_____

CHAPTER 7

Protection of Patients

OBJECTIVES

Upon completion of this chapter, the reader should be able to:

- Discuss the importance of immobilization of the patient during an X-ray exposure

- Describe beam-limiting apparatus and name the mechanism that best limits the X-ray beam

- Explain the purpose of X-ray beam filtration in diagnostic radiography

- State the reasons for using gonadal shielding during radiologic examinations and recognize the varieties of shields employed

- Discuss the necessity for using correct exposure factors for all radiologic procedures

- Demonstrate how the use of high-speed film-screen combinations decreases radiographic exposure to the patient

- Explain the rationale for decreasing the number of repeat radiographs

- Discuss how patient exposure may be reduced during fluoroscopic procedures

Notes: _____

IMMOBILIZATION

If there is patient movement during an X-ray exposure, there will be blurring of the radiographic image, and the radiologist will be unable to obtain an accurate diagnosis from such a film. The consequence of this would be a repeat exposure, resulting in twice the radiation to the patient and radiographer.

The need for repeat exposures can sometimes be the result of lack of communication between the patient and radiographer. The patient should be advised that a procedure may cause discomfort or possibly unusual feelings. A communication gap may occur as the result of insufficient or poorly interpreted instructions. Competent directions between the radiographer and the patient can help to prevent the need for repeat radiographs.

An example of this might be a barium enema exam. The radiographer should explain to the patient that there might be some minimal discomfort as the barium sulfate is administered into the colon, but that any discomfort will soon subside. The patient should be instructed that to avoid any possible repeat X-rays, it is necessary to try to control any **voluntary motion** during the study while experiencing any discomfort.

To reduce voluntary patient motion, the radiographer should use immobilization techniques during the radiation exposure. There are numerous products available for this purpose. These immobilization devices may be necessary when radiographing infants (Figure 7–1), and when examining patients who are incapacitated and thus unable to cooperate with the radiographer in not moving during the exposures.

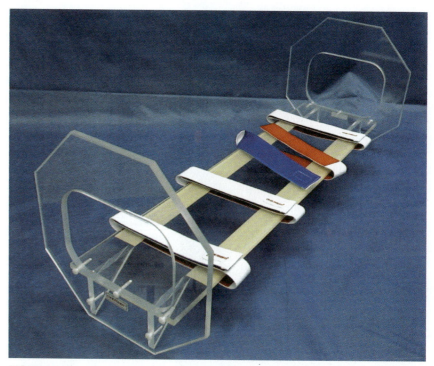

FIGURE 7–1
Infant immobilization cradle (Courtesy of Medi-inn Ltd.)

When dealing with **involuntary** patient **motion**, the radiographer should reduce radiation exposure times along with using immobilization mechanisms.

If the part being studied moves during the X-ray exposure, the result is motion unsharpness. Motion unsharpness can be restricted by using as short an exposure time possible.

Examples of involuntary patient motion would be heart contraction/relaxation and bowel peristalsis. The best way to reduce the chance of such involuntary patient motion is the use of minimal exposure times.

BEAM RESTRICTION

Scatter radiation is produced during a Compton interaction. In this interaction, a primary photon interacts with an outer-shell electron and changes direction, thereby becoming a scattered photon. Proper beam restriction will keep the total amount of tissue irradiation to a minimum and has great importance in both improving image quality and reducing patient dose.

As the beam is restricted, fewer primary photons are emitted from the tube and collimator and fewer scattered photons are created. Additionally, the decrease in the number of primary photons results in a decrease in the dose to the patient.

The principal factors that affect the amount of scatter produced are: 1) kilovoltage and 2) the irradiated material. In order to control the amount of scatter produced, it is important to understand how kilovoltage and the irradiated material affect scatter production.

Kilovoltage

Kilovoltage affects the penetrability of the beam. As kVp increases, fewer photons undergo interaction with matter and more pass through the patient to interact with the film. For the photons that undergo an interaction, the photoelectric absorption and Compton interactions are predominant in the diagnostic X-ray range. Although the total number of photons that undergo interaction decreases with increased kVp, a shift is seen in the percentage of photoelectric versus Compton interactions as kVp increases. As the kilovoltage increases, the percentage of X-rays that undergo a Compton interaction increases and the percentage of photons that undergo photoelectric absorption decreases. Because Compton interactions create scatter, as kilovoltage increases the percentage of primary photons that will undergo scattering also increases. At the same time, the percentage of primary photons that are absorbed photoelectrically decreases, resulting in a reduction in patient dose.

In radiography, the kilovoltage level is selected based predominantly on the size of the part being examined and the radiographic contrast desired for the image. When kilovoltage is increased without any other changes in technical factors, more scatter will result. If, however, the increase in kilovoltage is accompanied by a reduction in mAs to maintain the same dose, the overall result will be a decrease in the amount of scatter produced. Overall fewer photons are needed to create an acceptable image.

Irradiated Material

The amount of scatter created during an interaction is affected by the volume and atomic number of the material being irradiated. The volume of irradiated material is controlled by field size and patient thickness.

As the volume of irradiated tissue increases, the amount of scatter increases. Volume increases as the field size increases or as the patient thickness increases. Larger field sizes, such as with 14 × 17-inch (35 × 32-cm) film, allow for more photons to interact with tissue, thereby creating more scatter. Larger body parts have more tissue to interact with the photons, resulting in greater scatter production. In order to decrease scatter, the smallest possible field size should be used. It is for this reason that beam restriction is an important part of scatter reduction and, of course, patient protection.

BEAM-LIMITING DEVICES

Decreasing the area of the X-ray beam helps to reduce absorbed and scattered radiation by the patient. This is accomplished by using X-ray beam-limiting apparatus called diaphragms, **cones**, and collimators.

Aperture Diaphragms

The simplest type of **beam-limitation device** is the **aperture diaphragm**. It is a piece of flat lead containing a hole in its center. Attached to the tube head, it confines the X-ray beam so that a 1 cm unexposed border is visible on all sides of the finished radiograph (Figure 7–2). Aperture diaphragms are used in special procedure angiography studies.

Cones

Cones are circular metal structures that attach to the X-ray tube housing to restrict the X-ray beam to a predetermined circular size. They may be either a straight tube or a flared cylinder (Figure 7–3A and B). Cones are used for lateral *sella turcica* films, sinuses, L5/S-1 spine

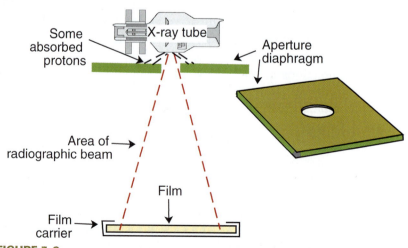

FIGURE 7–2
Aperture diaphragm

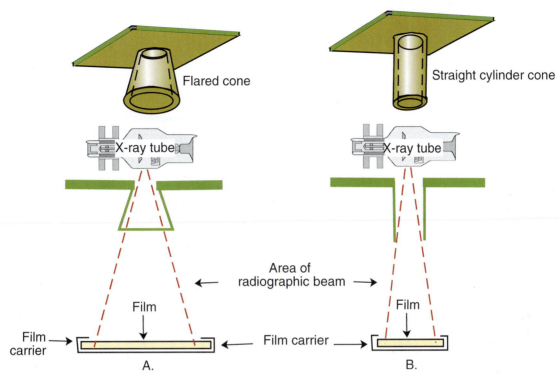

Flared cone

Straight cylinder cone

X-ray tube

X-ray tube

Area of
radiographic beam

Film

Film

Film
carrier

Film carrier

A.

B.

FIGURE 7–3A
Cones

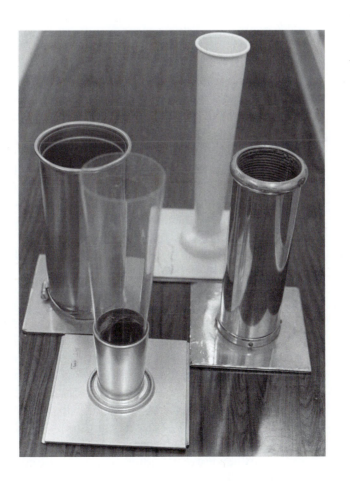

FIGURE 7–3B
Cones

Notes:

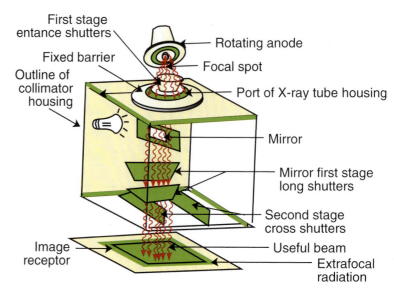

FIGURE 7–4
Reducing light field to area of clinical interest

radiographs, and dental radiography. The greatest beam limitation occurs with the longest cone and smallest diameter available. Metal and/or lead cones may also be used in dental radiography. The use of lead-lined cones results in the least exposure to the patient.

Collimators

The most broadly used beam-restricting device is the **variable-aperture collimator**, which is composed of an upper and lower pair of lead shutters. The shutters are at right angles to each other and move independently of the other pair (Figure 7–4). They may be adjusted to numerous square or rectangular field sizes. Variable shutter-type collimators also contain a lamp and a mirror. The lamp provides a light source to illuminate the area of interest, and the mirror is used to deflect the light toward the patient anatomy. A cross-hair in the light field marks the center of the X-ray beam. Collimators are the most widely used beam-restricting device because they contain a light source that helps the radiographer to correctly center the X-ray beam on the specific area to be radiographed. They also regulate the field size to the anatomical structure of interest. The purpose of the lead shutters is to restrict X-ray field size. The upper shutters absorb off-focus radiation before it leaves the X-ray tube. The lower shutters are mounted below the lamp and mirror, and further restrict the X-ray beam to the area of interest. Reducing the light field to only the area of clinical interest helps to reduce unnecessary patient exposure.

Equipment may be supplied with automatic collimation devices that are electronically interlocked with the Bucky tray so that the X-ray beam size is automatically restricted to the cassette size in use (Figure 7–5). Accuracy within 2% of the SID is required with automatic collimation devices (2% × 100 cm = 0.02 × 100 = 2 cm). When correctly adjusted, automatic collimation causes an unexposed border on all sides of the radiograph.

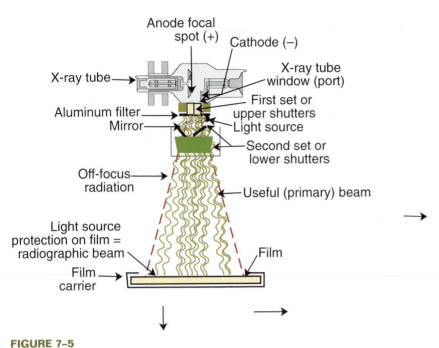

FIGURE 7–5
Unexposed border on all sides of radiograph

X-RAY BEAM FILTRATION

In conventional X-ray tubes, to assist in reducing patient exposure, an aluminum filter is inserted in the path of the X-ray beam. Filters absorb low energy photons, which improves the beam quality and increases average beam energy (hardness).

Because filtration absorbs some X-ray photons, it decreases the intensity of radiation. The photons not absorbed by the filtration are more penetrating and have less chance of being absorbed by the body. Thus, the patient-absorbed dose is decreased when correct filtration is placed in the X-ray beam path. If proper filtration is not used, low energy X-ray photons are absorbed by the body (Figure 7–6).

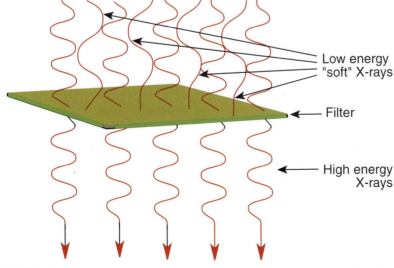

FIGURE 7–6
Filtration absorbing low energy photons

Notes:

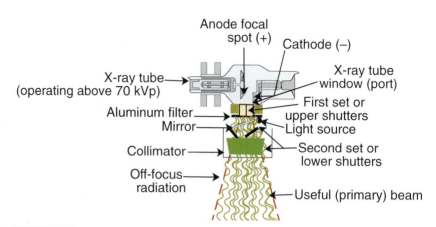

FIGURE 7–7
Filtration requirements for kVp levels

The two types of filtration are inherent and added. **Inherent filtration** consists of the glass window of the X-ray tube and the cooling oil surrounding the tube housing. **Added filtration** consists of aluminum or aluminum equivalent (Al eq.) of appropriate thickness inserted outside the glass window of the tube housing. The combination of inherent filtration plus added filtration equals **total filtration**. Inherent filtration increases as the tube ages.

The peak kilovoltage of an X-ray unit is the determining factor for the total filtration required (Figure 7–7).

Requirements for filtration in fixed radiographic equipment are:

Operating kVp	Minimum Total Filtration in mm Al eq.
Below 50	0.5
50–70	1.5
Above 70	2.5

The minimum total filtration for mobile diagnostic and/or fluoroscopic units is 2.5 mm Al eq.

To verify whether a diagnostic X-ray beam is adequately filtered, the **half-value layer (HVL)** of the beam must be measured. The HVL is the thickness of material that will reduce the X-ray intensity to half its original value. This measurement is obtained by quality control personnel on an annual basis, and also after repairs have been performed on the tube housing or collimator systems. The HVL is a characteristic of the X-ray beam and measures the beam quality.

An example of this would be to assume an original tube intensity of 100 mR. If one HVL is added, the new intensity would be 50 mR, or equal to one-half the original intensity. Table 7–1 shows the change in HVL with increase in kVp for fixed radiographic units having 2.5 mm Al total filtration.

GONADAL SHIELDING

The first step in providing gonad protection for a patient during an X-ray exposure is to properly collimate the X-ray beam to include only the area of clinical interest. Gonad shields should be used when

TABLE 7–1

Change in HVL with increase in kVp

kVp	HVL (mm Al)
50	1.9
75	2.8
100	3.7
125	4.6

Notes:

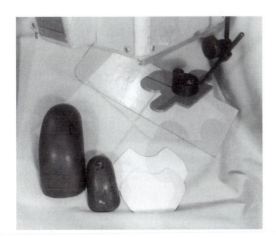

FIGURE 7–8
Gonadal shields

the gonads are in or within 5 cm of the primary X-ray beam (Figure 7–8). **Gonad shielding** should be utilized for anyone thought to be within the reproductive age. Gonadal shielding should not be used when it interferes with necessary diagnostic information.

Flat Contact Shields

Flat contact shields are composed of rubberized lead strips. These are laid directly over the patient's gonads, and may be secured to the patient with tape if necessary. These shields are useful for simple recumbent studies.

Shadow Shields

Shadow shields consist of a radiopaque material. This type of gonad shield is suspended from the X-ray tube housing, casting a shadow over the gonadal area. These shields are useful when encountering sterile fields such as in the operating room.

Shaped Contact Shields

Shaped contact shields consist of lead. These are worn by male patients, and are held in place by some type of disposable supporter. The shield is placed into a pouch inside the supporter. These shields are useful when doing oblique, lateral, and erect studies. They may be used during fluoroscopic stomach studies. It is rare to find these currently in use.

EXPOSURE AND TECHNIQUE FACTORS

The radiographer can significantly reduce the approximate entrance skin exposure to the patient by judicious selection of technique exposure factors. Studies have shown that over 50% of repeated exposures are the result of improper technical factor selection. Table 7–2 illustrates the effect each of the major technical factors has on patient dose. In most instances, when a technical factor is varied, other factors will be modified to maintain radiographic density. Therefore, the

TABLE 7-2

Effects of Radiographic Exposure Variables on Patient Dose

Variable	Variable Is Increased Compensation	Effect of Patient Dose When:	
		Variable Is Increased but Image Receptor Exposure Is Maintained by Compensating	
		with kVp Only	with mAs Only
Kilovoltage	+	NA	−
Milliamperage	+	+	0
Time	+	+	0
Distance			
SID	−	−	0
SOD	−	−	0
OID	+	+	+
Focal spot size	0	NA	NA
Filtration	−	−	+
Field size	+	varies	varies
Gonadal shielding	−	NA	NA
Subject part density	+	+	+
Grid ratio	0	+	+
Intensifying screens	0	−	−
Film speed	0	−	−
Film processing			
Developer time	0	−	−
Developer temperature	0	−	−
Developer replenishment	0	−	−

From Carlton, R., & Adler, A. (2006). *Principles of radiographic imaging: An art and science* (4th ed.). Clifton Park, NY: Thomson Delmar Learning.

Notes:

important information is not the direct result of the technical factor change, but the result of compensation to maintain radiographic density or other components of image quality.

Kilovoltage Range

When kVp is increased without compensating for other factors, patient dose is increased. Therefore, a decrease in kVp is desired when attempting to reduce patient dose. However, when an increase in kVp is compensated for by a decrease in mAs to maintain radiographic density, a significant reduction in patient dose is achieved. Selection of the highest possible kilovoltage consistent with image quality is the best method of using exposure factors to reduce patient dose. With fixed kilovoltage systems, care must be taken to achieve an optimal kVp that is within acceptance limits. Because fixed kVp technique systems tend to utilize higher optimal kVp levels, they usually reduce patient entrance skin exposures.

Remember that generator phase also has an effect on kilovoltage output. Although an increase in the number of pulses from the generator would seem to increase the patient dose because of the increased average photon energy, there is actually a substantial decrease in patient ESE (from 40 to 6%) because of the decrease in the percentage of lower energy photons from the X-ray tube. The lower energy photons tend to be absorbed in the body instead of being transmitted to the image receptor, thus contributing to patient ESE without adding any information to the image receptor.

Milliamperage and Time

When mAs is decreased, patient dose is also decreased. When an increase in mAs is compensated by a decrease in kVp, patient dose will increase. An inverse relationship exists between mAs and kVp in maintaining radiographic density. To decrease patient dose, mAs should be maintained at the lowest possible level because there is a direct relationship between mAs and exposure. Because variable kVp technique systems tend to utilize lower kVp levels with higher mAs, the result can be higher average patient ESE than with fixed kVp systems.

The use of high kVp and low mAs will result in reducing the absorbed dose to the patient (Figure 7–9). The technique selected

A.

High kVp, low mAs

B.

Low kVp, high mAs

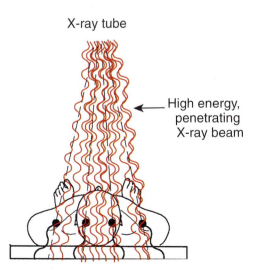
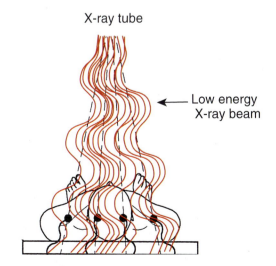

FIGURE 7–9

Use of high kVp and low mAs to reduce absorbed dose

should provide adequate part penetration, acceptable film density, and proper radiographic contrast.

FILM-SCREEN CONSIDERATIONS

A significant reduction in patient exposure results from using the highest speed **intensifying screens** and films consistent with satisfactory image quality. An example of this would be use of high-speed intensifying screens and films during GI studies.

> **EXAMPLE**
>
> A lateral skull X-ray is taken at 65 kVp and 50 mAs, which results in a skin dose of 300 mrad. If the kVp is increased to 75 (a 15% increase), and the mAs is reduced by 1/2, to 25 mAs, the radiographic density should remain the same. (This technique adjustment would cause an increase in exposure latitude, and a decrease in contrast.) What is the patient skin dose? Answer:
>
> $$Dose = (300 \text{ mrad})(25mAs/50mAs)(75kVp/65kVp) = (300 \text{ mrad})$$
> $$(0.5)(1.33) = 200 \text{ mrad}$$
>
> (Caution should be taken when kVp is decreased and mAs increased, as there may not be adequate penetration using the new lower kVp).

Radiographic Film

Film is constructed at different speeds for use with intensifying screens that enhance the action of X-rays. Film speed influences radiographic exposure time. Increasing film speed means less exposure is required to obtain an image. With this decrease in exposure, there is a decrease in patient dose.

Intensifying Screens

Intensifying screens accelerate the action of X-rays by converting X-ray energy into visible light. Because a single X-ray photon can produce 80–95 light photons from an intensifying screen, this conversion speeds up the film exposure process. Approximately 95% of the density of a recorded image results from the visible light photons emitted by the intensifying screens. Because more light is emitted from the screens, radiographic exposure can be reduced. This leads to a reduction in patient dose.

Rare-earth intensifying screens are more efficient than calcium-tungstate intensifying screens in converting X-ray energy photons into light photons. The rare-earth screens absorb three to five times more X-ray energy than calcium-tungstate screens, thereby emitting more light. Rare-earth screens are from two to ten times faster than calcium-tungstate screens. This increase in speed significantly reduces patient dose. Rare-earth screens are widely used in GI radiography.

Kilovoltage affects screen speed. As kVp increases, screen speed increases. This results in a reduction in patient dose.

ELECTRONIC IMAGING

While traditional projection radiography, which uses film/screen imaging, is still utilized, many imaging departments are converting to **electronic imaging**. Electronic imaging includes **computed radiography (CR)** and **digital radiography (DR)**. Although X-ray photons are still required to produce electronic images, CR and DR use computers to create, read, and process, display and manipulate, and store those images.

Computed Radiography (CR)

The fundamental difference between computed radiography and conventional analog imaging is the replacement of film-screens with photostimulable phosphor plates. These digital plates require a plate reader, a port of linkage to patient text data, and connection to an output device such as a printer or a picture archiving communication systems (PACS) network. The technologists need a CR imaging system that includes storage phosphor cassettes, a storage phosphor reader, bar code scanner, remote operator panel for entering patient data, and a clinical workstation for reviewing and printing from PACS.

The basic component of CR image capture is the photostimulable phosphor cassette. The phosphors used to coat the screen are europium-activated barium fluorohalide crystals. The phosphors in these screens fluoresce upon exposure to ionizing radiation emitted from the X-ray tube. Radiation energy causes the phosphors to fluoresce, releasing a high fraction of the absorbed energy from the screens. Remnant energy is stored in the phosphors as a latent image. It is the stored energy in the form of a latent image that is used to produce the CR image, but the image must be released from the phosphors and further processed. When stimulated with infrared or white light, photostimulable phosphors release light proportional to the stored energy, which can be detected by a photomultiplier tube(s) as an image signal. Latent images can be kept on a plate for up to 8 hours.

The dynamic range of exposure for photostimulable phosphors is linear over a range of greater than 10,000 to 1, whereas for analog radiographic images produced by screens it is roughly 40 to 1. Over-exposure or under-exposure of radiographic images seen in conventional film-screen imaging is virtually eliminated by photostimulable phosphor technology imaging.

CR affords much larger exposure latitude as compared to conventional projection radiography. Mistakes in exposure selection can be virtually eliminated. Over-exposures of up to 500%, and under-exposures up to 80% are recoverable, thus eliminating the need for retakes. The same exposure factors as used with conventional screen/film systems are normally utilized for CR.

The use of CR allows for continued use of existing equipment. CR can also be used for mobile exams, tabletop exposures, and horizontal beam work.

Digital Radiography (DR)

Digital radiography does not use cassettes or the traditional X-ray table, as used in CR. Instead, it utilizes a direct capture system, which consists of solid state detector plates as the image receptor. These receptors are composed of barium fluorohalide compounds.

The solid state receptors convert X-ray photons into electrical energy. The two types of detectors utilized include either an indirect conversion flat panel detector or a charge coupled device (CCD) detector. These detectors use photostimulable phosphors that convert visible light into electrical energy. An analog to digital converter (ADC) next converts the analog image to a digital image, which can be viewed on a monitor in just a matter of seconds.

A second method of converting the X-ray photons into electrical energy utilizes a direct conversion flat panel detector. It contains a silicon layer that becomes electrically charged when exposed to X-rays. The electrical charge is then sent to the ADC for conversion to the digital image.

PATIENT POSITIONING

An effective method of reducing patient dose is through accurate and effective positioning. Avoidance of repeated exposures far outweighs all other methods. However, once positioning skills have been developed to a degree of competence, several positioning details may further reduce the total dose.

Some organs are especially sensitive to the effects of radiation, for example, the female breast, the kidneys, and the lens of the eye. Increased recorded detail and decreased distortion result when the area of interest is placed as close to the image receptor as possible. In most instances, a significant reduction in the total dose is achieved because this positioning also places the organ as far from the entrance exposure as possible.

GRIDS

Radiographic grids are placed between the patient and the image receptor to preferentially absorb scatter radiation. Because grids absorb primary as well as scatter radiation, technical factors must be increased to produce an image of acceptable film density. This increase in technical factors results in an increase in patient dose but image quality is significantly improved. The lowest possible grid ratio consistent with effective scatter removal should be utilized to keep patient dose as low as reasonably achievable.

THE PREGNANT PATIENT

To minimize the possible exposure to an embryo in the earliest days of a pregnancy, a guideline known as the 10-day rule was recommended by a number of advisory agencies. This guideline stated that elective abdominal X-ray examinations of fertile women should be postponed until the 10-day period following the onset of menstruation as it would be improbable that a woman would be pregnant during these days. Based on the current understanding of radiobiology, this rule is now considered obsolete, primarily because the egg for the next cycle reaches maximum sensitivity during the 10-day period. The application of this guideline within the radiology department has always proven difficult.

It is now the general belief that postponement of abdominal X-ray examinations is not necessary when the physician requesting the examination has considered the entire clinical state of the patient, including the possibility of pregnancy. The potential pregnancy status of all female patients of childbearing age should always be determined; in the event of known pregnancy, steps should be taken to minimize exposure to the fetus. One way to ensure against irradiating a woman in the early stages of pregnancy is to institute elective scheduling for nonemergency procedures. In many departments, female patients of childbearing ages are asked to provide the date of their last menstrual period (LMP). If there is a concern about a possible pregnancy, the patient's exam may be rescheduled. If a radiologic exam on a pregnant patient is deemed necessary, a diagnostic radiological physicist should perform calculations to estimate the actual fetal dose.

REPEAT RADIOGRAPHS

Repeat radiographs, which range from approximately 5–15%, result in additional patient exposure. Repeat examinations resulting from carelessness or poor radiographer judgment must be eliminated. The radiographer should select correct radiographic techniques and exposure factors that ensure high-quality radiographs.

Causes of repeat radiographs also include dirty screens, incorrectly loaded cassettes, light leaks, chemical fog, processor artifacts, incorrect projections, positioning errors, grid errors, and multiple exposures.

FLUOROSCOPIC PROCEDURES

Fluoroscopy produces the greatest patient radiation exposure in diagnostic radiology. Because X-ray exposures produce cumulative effects, the physician should evaluate the necessity of the exam. If the physician judges the exam necessary, precautions must be taken to minimize patient dose.

Image Intensification Fluoroscopy

This system converts the X-ray into an amplified visible light pattern. Image brightness increases approximately 7,000–20,000 times with **image intensification fluoroscopy**, as compared to conventional fluoroscopic systems. With the use of image intensified fluoroscopy,

Notes:

Notes:

the radiologist does not need to go through dark adaptation, as was necessary with conventional fluoroscopy. This increase in image brightness results in the use of less mA (approximately 1.5–2 mA for image intensification systems, as compared to 3–5 mA for conventional fluoroscopy). The consequent decrease in exposure rate results in a reduction in dose for the patient.

Intermittent/Pulsed Fluoroscopy The radiologist should use **intermittent or pulsed fluoroscopy** to decrease patient exposure and prolong tube life. This means that the radiologist should periodically activate the fluoroscopic tube, rather than having the tube continuously activated.

Limitation of Field Size Limitation of field size is accomplished by placing lead collimating shutters between the fluoroscopic tube and the patient. The fluoroscopic beam must be restricted to the smallest field that includes the area of interest, which reduces exposure to both patient and personnel. The radiologist should collimate to only the area of interest. Federal law prohibits the useful beam at the image receptor from exceeding the visible image area by more than 3% of the **source-image receptor distance (SID)**.

Exposure Factors The recommended operating factors are 90–100 kVp, 2–3 mA, and 2.5 mm Al equivalent filter for image intensified fluoroscopy. According to federal law, the source-tabletop distance must be at least 15 inches (38 cm) with stationary and 12 inches (30 cm) with mobile fluoroscopic equipment. Fluoroscopic exposure factors for pediatric patients necessitate a decrease in kVp by as much as 25%. The chosen kVp depends on thickness of part, the same as it does during conventional radiography.

A **cumulative timing device** must be furnished and used with all fluoroscopic units. This device is provided to preset the on-time of the fluoroscopic tube for a cumulative total of no more than five minutes. An audible signal will sound when five minutes has accumulated, and will continue to sound until the timer is reset to five minutes.

According to federal code, the exposure rate at the tabletop must be no greater than 10 R/min for fluoroscopic equipment with intensified fluoroscopic units and no greater than 5 R/min without intensified fluoroscopic units.

KEY CONCEPTS

- It is important to keep the patient immobilized to avoid artifact in the X-ray and to avoid repeat exposures.
- Beam limiting apparatus serve to control the direction of the beam to specific areas of the body. Collimators are the best device for this purpose.
- X-ray beam filtration reduces patient exposure by use of a filter to absorb low energy photons.

- It is important to use gonadal shielding to protect the patient's reproductive organs from radiation exposure. There are several varieties of shields used: flat contact shields, shadow shields, and shaped contact shields.
- Use of correct exposure factors limits the need for repeat exposures; factors to consider are high kVp and low mAs and high speed intensifying screens.
- Use of high speed intensifying screens converts X-ray energy into visible light, thus reducing the exposure of the patient to radiation.
- Reducing the number of repeat radiographs reduces the radiation exposure of both the patient and the radiographer.
- Radiation exposure during fluoroscopic procedures can be limited by using intermittent fluoroscopy and reducing the size of the exposed field.

Notes:

REVIEW QUESTIONS & EXERCISES
Crossword Puzzle

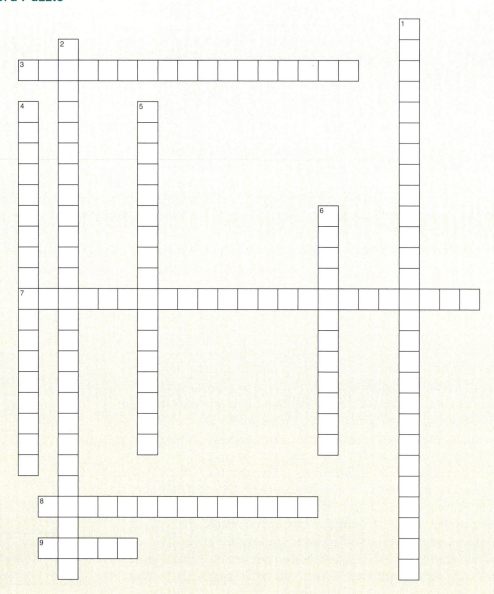

Across

3. Rubberized lead strips that are placed over areas of the body to protect them from exposure.

7. The procedure of periodically activating the flouro tube rather the having the tube continuously activated, thus reducing patient exposure and prolonging the life of the tube.

8. The thickness of the material that will reduce the X-ray intensity to half of its original value.

9. A circular metal structure attached to the X-ray tube housing to restrict the X-ray beam to a predetermined size.

Down

1. The area from the point of contact on the patient to the tube.

2. A pair of upper and lower level lead shutters at right angles to each other that can be adjusted to limit the size field the X-ray beam will expose.

4. Limiting the X-ray beam by use of a glass window in the tube and cooling oil surrounding the tube housing.

5. A piece of flat lead with a hole in the center that attaches to the X-ray tube to confine the area of the beam.

6. A radiopaque material that is suspended from the tube housing that casts a shadow over the area that should not be exposed.

Matching

Match the definition in the right column with the correct term from the left column.

_____ 1. Added filtration

_____ 2. Beam limitation device

_____ 3. Cumulative timing device

_____ 4. Gonad shielding

_____ 5. Image intensification fluoroscopy

_____ 6. Intensifying screen

_____ 7. Involuntary motion

_____ 8. Shaped contact shield

_____ 9. Total filtration

_____ 10. Voluntary motion

a. Lead devices that are shaped to fit over anatomical areas of the body to protect them from radiation exposure

b. The maximum amount of limitation of the X-ray beam through the use of both added and inherent filtration methods

c. Movement controlled by the patient

d. Protection of the reproductive organs from radiation exposure

e. A procedure used to increase the brightness of an image with a decreased exposure time

f. A device that serves to accelerate the action of X-rays by converting X-ray energy into visible light

g. Movement of the patient that is beyond the patient's control

h. Limiting the X-ray beam by the use of a piece of aluminum or aluminum equivalent outside the glass window of the housing tube

i. Equipment that reduces the beam to only those areas in need of exposure

j. A device that presets the on time for the tube to only 5-minute increments

Multiple Choice

1. In order to reduce the possibility of voluntary patient motion, the radiographer should:
   a. use an immobilization device.
   b. reduce radiation exposure time.
   c. disregard any communication with patient.
   d. use slow speed screens.

2. Which of the following is the most versatile type of X-ray beam limitation device?
   a. aperture diaphragm   c. cylinder
   b. cone   d. collimator

3. The function of filtration in diagnostic radiology is to:
   a. decrease short wavelength radiation, thus increasing patient skin dose.
   b. increase beam hardness, thus increasing patient skin dose.
   c. increase beam hardness, thus reducing patient skin dose.
   d. decrease beam hardness, thus reducing patient skin dose.

4. Which of the following combinations would reduce patient radiation dose during an X-ray examination?
   a. higher kVp, lower mAs, increased filtration
   b. lower kVp, higher mAs, decreased filtration
   c. higher kVp, higher mAs, decreased filtration
   d. lower kVp, lower mAs, increased filtration

5. Patient dose decreases when:
   a. high-speed radiographic film is used in combination with high-speed intensifying screens.
   b. rare-earth intensifying screens are not used.
   c. low kVp techniques are used.
   d. nonscreen film is used.

6. Repeat radiographs result in:
   a. no additional exposure to the patient.
   b. a double exposure of radiation to the patient.
   c. increased patient flow.
   d. increased productivity.

7. The source-tabletop distance must not be less than _____ for fixed fluoroscopes and not less than _____ for mobile fluoroscopes.
   a. 12 inches (30 cm), 6 inches (15 cm)
   b. 15 inches (38 cm), 12 inches (30 cm)
   c. 15 inches (38 cm), 9 inches (23 cm)
   d. 18 inches (45 cm), 15 inches (38 cm)

SITUATIONAL JUDGMENT TESTING

A barium enema has been ordered for your patient. You are concerned about voluntary patient motion. What would you do to best minimize the chance for this occurring during the exam?
   a. Use immobilization techniques.
   b. Utilize competent directions and communication between yourself and your patient.
   c. Utilize short exposure times.
   d. Utilize short exposure times along with using immobilization mechanisms.

EXPLORING THE WEB

1. Search the Web for additional information on patient safety during radiographic procedures. Can you find any information to hand out to patients? Are you able to find any additional tips to ensure the safety of your patients?

    _____

    _____

    _____

    _____

2. Search the Web for manufacturers of shielding equipment for use during radiographic procedures. List the pros and cons of the various types of equipment available. Are there any new technologies available to aid in patient protection and safety?

    _____

    _____

    _____

    _____

3. Search the Web for tips and techniques in working with children who are undergoing radiographic procedures. Are there any special circumstances to be aware of with this population? How can you gain a child's trust? How can you help the child understand what the machinery will do?

    _____

    _____

    _____

    _____

CASE STUDY

You are about to X-ray a patient who is exhibiting voluntary motion. Discuss what steps you would take to minimize this motion. Compare this with involuntary motion.

_____

_____

_____

_____

_____

SECTION 3 REVIEW

MULTIPLE CHOICE

1. How tall must primary protective barriers be?
   a. 3 feet
   b. 4 feet
   c. 7 feet
   d. 10 feet

2. Leakage radiation from the X-ray tube housing shall not exceed _____ at a distance of 1 meter from the tube.
   a. 1 mR/hr
   b. 10 mR/hr
   c. 100 mR/hr
   d. 1,000 mR/hr

3. The minimum lead equivalency of a lead apron must be at least:
   a. 0.12 mm
   b. 0.25 mm
   c. 0.5 mm
   d. 1 mm

4. How many rems of whole-body cumulative exposure would a 45-year-old radiographer be allowed to receive?
   a. 15
   b. 45
   c. 35
   d. 25

5. A protective lead curtain that is at least _____ Pb equivalent must be positioned between the patient and the fluoroscopy operator.
   a. 0.025 mm
   b. 0.25 mm
   c. 2.5 mm
   d. 25 mm

6. The function of a filter is to remove which of the following from the X-ray beam?
   a. low energy photons
   b. high energy photons
   c. secondary radiation
   d. scattered radiation

7. Which of the following is the best type of gonadal shielding to use during a sterile field procedure?
   a. flat contact shields
   b. shadow shields
   c. shaped contact shields
   d. lead sheet

8. A fluoroscope must be equipped with a cumulative timing device that times the radiation exposure and sounds an audible alarm after the fluoroscope has been energized for:
   a. 1 minute.
   b. 2 minutes.
   c. 3 minutes.
   d. 5 minutes.

9. Which of the following is not a type of beam limitation device?
   a. collimator
   b. cone
   c. filter
   d. aperture diaphragm

10. The minimum source to tabletop distance permitted in mobile fluoroscopy is:
    a. 4 inches.
    b. 9 inches.
    c. 12 inches.
    d. 15 inches.

11. The effective dose-equivalent limit to the lens of the eye for a radiographer is:
    a. 1 rem.
    b. 5 rem.
    c. 10 rem.
    d. 15 rem.

12. Student radiographers under the age of 18 have an effective dose-equivalent limit of:
    a. 0.1 rem.
    b. 0.5 rem.
    c. 1 rem.
    d. 5 rem.

13. The total effective dose-equivalent limit to the fetus of a pregnant radiographer is:
    a. 0.1 rem.
    c. 1 rem.
    b. 0.5 rem.
    d. 5 rem.

14. Secondary protective barriers must have a lead thickness of:
    a. 1/64 inch.
    c. 1/16 inch.
    b. 1/32 inch.
    d. 1/4 inch.

15. The intensity of scattered radiation at 1 meter from the patient as compared to the intensity at the patient is:
    a. 0.001%.
    c. 0.1%.
    b. 0.01%.
    d. 1%.

16. The _____ is the percentage of time that the X-ray beam is energized and directed toward a particular wall.
    a. occupancy factor (T)
    c. workload (W)
    b. use factor (U)
    d. tube on-time (TO)

17. In order to obey radiation safety regulations, what must the fluoroscopic exposure switch do?
    a. Abort fluoroscopic exposure after 5 minutes.
    b. Be at the end of a 6-foot long expandable cord.
    c. Make an audible sound during fluoroscopic exposure.
    d. Be of the deadman type.

18. In mobile fluoroscopy, the source-to-tabletop distance must not be less than _____.
    a. 6 inches
    c. 15 inches
    b. 12 inches
    d. 20 inches

19. If the exposure rate to a radiographer positioned 3 feet from a radiation source is 8 mR/min, what will be the dose to the radiographer at a distance of 6 feet from the source?
    a. 1 mR/min
    c. 16 mR/min
    b. 2 mR/min
    d. 32 mR/min

20. The exposure rate to a radiographer 3 feet from a radiation source is 40 R/hr. What distance from the source is necessary to decrease the exposure to 10 R/hr?
    a. 1 feet
    c. 6 feet
    b. 2 feet
    d. 12 feet

21. Radiation monitoring of personnel is required when personnel receive _____ % of the annual effective dose-equivalent limit.
    a. 0.01
    c. 5
    b. 1
    d. 10

22. By what factor does a thyroid shield reduce radiation dose?
    a. 10
    b. 4
    b. 7
    d. 1

23. If an original intensity was 300 mR, and mAs is increased from 20 to 40 mAs, what would be the new intensity?
    a. 150 mAs
    b. 600 mAs
    b. 300 mAs
    d. 900 mAs

24. If 70 kVp produces an intensity of 200 mR, what will be the intensity at 100 kVp if no other factors are changed?
    a. 100
    b. 408
    b. 300
    d. 808

25. Voluntary patient motion is best reduced by utilizing:
    a. long exposure times.   c. immobilization devices.
    b. low mA.   d. high kVp.

26. To within what percent of the SID must the collimator light and actual irradiated area be accurate?
    a. 2%   c. 10%
    b. 5%   d. 22%

27. The greatest beam limitation is accomplished when the cone/cylinder is _____ and the diameter opening is _____.
    a. shorter, bigger   c. longer, bigger
    b. shorter, smaller   d. longer, smaller

28. How much total filtration is required when using over 70 kVp?
    a. 1.5 mm Al   c. 3.0 mm Al
    b. 2.5 mm Al   d. 4.0 mm Al

29. Which of the following exposure techniques will provide the least amount of radiation exposure to the patient?
    a. 50 mAs, 90 kVp   c. 200 mAs, 50 kVp
    b. 100 mAs, 90 kVp   d. 400 mAs, 50 kVp

30. Which of the following will best reduce radiation exposure to the patient?
    a. Use non-screen film.   c. Decrease kVp.
    b. Use rare-earth screens.   d. Increase mAs.

31. The number of repeat radiographs can be reduced by:
    a. disregarding communication between patient and radiographer.
    b. eliminating voluntary patient motion by using short exposure times.
    c. eliminating involuntary patient motion by using immobilization devices.
    d. eliminating voluntary patient motion by using immobilization devices.

32. A fluoroscope must be equipped with a cumulative timing device that times the radiation exposure and sounds an audible alarm after the fluoroscope has been energized for:
    a. 1 minute.   c. 3 minutes.
    b. 2 minutes.   d. 5 minutes.

33. Which of the following is not a type of beam-limitation device?
    a. collimator   c. filter
    b. cone   d. aperture diaphragm

34. The focal spot-to-table distance in fixed fluoroscopy must be
    a. a minimum of 7 inches.   c. a minimum of 15 inches.
    b. a minimum of 12 inches. d. a maximum of 12 inches.

35. Half-value layer (HVL) is defined as the thickness of a designated absorber required to:
    a. decrease the intensity of the primary beam by 50% of its initial value.
    b. decrease the intensity of the primary beam by 25% of its initial value.
    c. increase the intensity of the primary beam by 50% of its initial value.
    d. increase the intensity of the primary beam by 25% of its initial value.

Bibliography

American College of Radiology. 1985. *Medical radiation: A guide to good practice.* Chicago, IL: American College of Radiology.

American Registry of Radiologic Technologists. 2008. *Certification handbook: Radiography, nuclear medicine technology, radiation therapy technology.* St. Paul, MN: ARRT.

American Society of Radiologic Technologists. 2007. *Radiography curriculum.* Albuquerque, NM: ASRT.

Bushberg, J., J. Seibert, E. Leidholdt, and J. Boone. 2001. *The essential physics of medical imaging.* 2nd ed. Baltimore: Lippincott, Williams and Wilkins.

Bushong, S. 1997. *Radiologic science for technologists.* 6th ed. St. Louis, MO: Mosby.

Callaway, W. 2006. *Mosby's comprehensive review of radiography.* 4th ed. St. Louis, MO: Mosby.

Carlton, R., and A. Adler, 2006. *Principles of radiographic imaging: An art and a science.* 4th ed., Clifton Park, NY: Delmar, Cengage Learning.

Committee on Biological Effects of Ionizing Radiation. 1989. *BEIR V report. The health effects of exposure to low levels of ionizing radiation.* Washington: National Academy Press.

Curry, T., J. Dowdey, and R. Murry. 1990. *Christensen's physics of diagnostic radiology.* 4th ed. Baltimore: Lippincott, Williams and Wilkins.

Dekaban, A. 1968. Abnormalities in children exposed to x-radiation during various stages of gestation: Tentative timetable of radiation injury to the human fetus. *Journal of nuclear medicine,* 9:471–477.

Dowd, S., and E. Tilson. 1999. *Practical radiation protection and applied radiobiology.* 2nd ed. Philadelphia: Saunders.

Gurley, L., and W. Callaway. 2006. *Introduction to radiologic technology.* 6th ed. St. Louis, MO: Mosby.

Hall, E., and A. Giaccia. 2006. *Radiobiology for the radiologist.* 6th ed. Baltimore: Lippincott, Williams and Wilkins.

Hendee, W., and R. Ritenour. 2002. *Medical imaging physics.* 4th ed. New York: Wiley-Liss.

Hubner, K., and S. Fry, eds. 1980. *The medical basis for radiation accident preparedness,* New York: Elsevier.

International Commission of Radiologic Protection. 1991. 1990 recommendations of the ICRP. *ICRP Publication 60.* Elmsford, NY: Pergamon Press.

Martin, J. 2006. *Physics for radiation protection.* 2nd ed. New York: Wiley-VCH.

Martin, J., and C. Lee. 2003. *Principles of radiological health and safety.* New York: Wiley.

National Council on Radiation Protection and Measurements. 1989. Medical X-ray, electron beam and gamma-ray protection for energies up to MeV. *NCRP Report No. 102.* Bethesda, MD: NCRP.

National Council on Radiation Protection and Measurements. 1989. Radiation protection for medical and allied health personnel. *NCRP Report No. 105.* Bethesda, MD: NCRP.

National Council on Radiation Protection and Measurements. 1993. Limitation of exposure to ionizing radiation. *NCRP Report No. 116.* Bethesda, MD: NCRP.

Pizarello, D., and R. Witcofski. 1982. *Medical radiation biology.* 2nd ed. Philadelphia, PA: Lea and Febiger.

Radiation Effects Research Foundation. 1976. *Technical Report RERF 10–76.*

Saia, D. 2006. *Radiography PREP.* 4th ed. New York: McGraw Hill.

Saia, D. 2006. *Lange Q and A for the radiography examination.* 6th ed. New York: McGraw Hill.

Scott, A., E. Fong. 2003. *Body structures and functions.* 10th ed., Clifton Park, NY: Delmar, Cengage Learning.

Seeram, E. 2001. *Rad tech's guide to radiation protection.* Wiley-Blackwell.

Selman, J. 1985. *The fundamentals of X-ray and radium physics.* 7th ed. Springfield, IL: Thomas.

Selman, J. 2000. *The fundamentals of imaging physics and radiobiology.* 9th ed. Springfield, IL: Thomas.

Statkiewicz-Sherer, M., P. Visconti, and E. Ritenour. 2006. *Radiation protection in medical radiography.* 5th ed. St. Louis, MO: Mosby.

Thompson, M., M. Hattaway, J. Hall, and S. Dowd. 1994. *Principles of imaging science and protection.* Philadelphia: Saunders.

Tortora, G., and B. Dickinson. 2006. *Principles of anatomy and physiology.* 11th ed. New York: Wiley.

Travis, E. 2000. *Primer of medical radiobiology.* 2nd ed. St. Louis, MO: Mosby.

U.S. Nuclear Regulatory Commission. 1987. Instruction concerning prenatal radiation exposure. *NRC Regulatory Guide* 8:13, Rev. 2.

Wagner, L., and L. Hayman. 1982. "Pregnancy in women radiologists." *Radiology, 145:* 599–562.

Glossary

A

Aberration Imperfection.

Absolute risk model (1) Estimates a continual increase in risk, independent of the age-specific cancer risk at time of exposure; also known as the additive risk model. (2) number of cases per one million persons per rad per year.

Acentric On the outside; the periphery.

Acute Rapid, severe.

Added filtration Limiting the X-ray beam by the use of a piece of aluminum or aluminum equivalent outside the glass window of the housing tube.

Agreement states Those states that have agreements with the Nuclear Regulatory Commission to take responsibility to enforce radiation protection guidelines through the states' department of health.

ALARA As low as reasonably achievable.

Alopecia Hair loss.

Amino acid An organic compound that is the building block of proteins and the end product of protein digestion.

Anabolism The construction phase of metabolism, when a cell takes the substances from blood that are necessary for repair and growth and converts them into cytoplasm. The opposite of catabolism.

Anaphase A stage in mitosis and meiosis between metaphase and telophase in which chromatids migrate toward opposite poles of the cell.

Anemia Reduction in red blood cell counts.

Ankylosing spondylitis Immobility of the vertebrae.

Anomaly Departure from normal.

Aperture diaphragm A piece of flat lead with a hole in the center. This equipment is attached to the tube to confine the X-ray beam to the area of the hole. All areas surrounding the hole will remain unexposed.

Atrophy Shrinking.

Autosomes Any chromosome that is other than the sex (X and Y) chromosomes.

B

Beam-limitation device Equipment that reduces the beam to only those areas in need of exposure; all other areas will not be exposed to the beam.

BEIR Committee on the Biological Effects of Ionizing Radiation.

Benign Nonprogressive.

Bone marrow dose A measure of the radiation that has been absorbed into the patient's bone marrow.

Bystander effect The effect of radiation on cells that are adjacent to those directly affected by radiation.

C

Carcinogenic Cancer-causing.

Carcinoma A growth or tumor.

Catabolism The destructive phase of metabolism, in which complex substances are changed into simpler substances. The opposite of anabolism.

Centromere The constricted area of the chromosome that separates the chromosome into two arms.

Chromatid The halves into which the chromosome is longitudinally divided, which are held together by the centromere and move to opposite poles of a dividing cell during anaphase.

Chromatin A material in the nucleus that contains genetic information. It is DNA that is joined to a protein structure base.

Chromosome The linear thread of a cell nucleus. They contain DNA, which makes up genes, our hereditary blueprint.

Chronic Slow, progressive.

Computed radiography Radiography using a solid-state imaging device, such as a photostimulable phosphor plate, and recovering, enhancing, and displaying the image using a digital computer.

Cones A circular metal structure attached to the X-ray tube housing to restrict the X-ray beam to a predetermined size.

Controlled area An area occupied by radiation personnel.

Crypts of Lieberkuhn Radiosensitive cells that are a precursor to the population of villi cells.

Cumulative timing device A device that presets the on time for the tube to only 5-minute increments.

Cytopenia Depression of all blood cell counts.

D

Deadman type Exposure control switch that is either a foot pedal or a hand switch.

Deletion A chromosomal effect that causes a loss of genetic material.

Deoxyribonucleic acid (DNA) A polymer composed of deoxyribonucleotides. Arranged in a double helix, it is present in chromosomes in the cell's nucleus, and is the carrier of genetic information.

Dermis Middle layer of the skin.

Desquamation Peeling skin.

Dicentric A chromosome that has two centers or two centromeres.

Digital radiography A form of X-ray imaging where digital X-ray sensors are used instead of traditional photographic film.

Diploid Possessing two sets of chromosomes, in reference to somatic cells, which have two times the number of chromosomes present in the egg or sperm. Referred to as 2n; in humans, the 2n or diploid number = 46.

Direct effect A result of ionization and excitation, an interaction that happens directly on a critical biologic macromolecule.

Division delay Slow-down of cell division due to irradiation.

DNA proofreading A system that checks newly synthesized DNA for errors and corrects them when they are found.

Dose Amount of radiation exposure.

Dose-response relationship (curve) A graphical representation of observed effects (response) compared with radiation dose.

Dosimetry Measurement of ionizing radiation doses to personnel.

Doubling dose The dose of radiation required per generation to double the spontaneous mutation rate.

Duplication A chromosome mutation in which either one or both segments of a chromosome join to another chromosome.

E

Early effect of radiation The response of human cells exposed to radiation within minutes, days, or weeks of exposure.

Edema Swelling.

Effective dose limit The lowest dose of radiation that will maintain health with no ill effects.

Electronic imaging Technology that utilizes computed and digital radiography.

Entrance skin exposure (ESE) A measure of the radiation to the patient's skin at the skin entrance surface; also known as the skin dose.

Enzyme A complex organic protein which accelerates chemical reactions.

Epidermis Outer layer of the skin.

Epilation Hair loss.

Erythema Reddening of skin.

Erythroblasts Precursors for red blood cells.

Excess risk The number of excess cases of cancer observed compared with expected spontaneous occurrence.

F

Fibrosis Abnormal formation of fibrous tissue.

Film badge A type of dosimeter consisting of radiation dosimetry film to determine the amount of exposure personnel have received.

Flat contact shield Rubberized lead strips that are placed over areas of the body to protect them from exposure.

Follicle Sac or cavity.

Follicular Sac- or cavity-like.

Fractionation The splitting of radiation into smaller amounts over a period of time.

Free radical An atom that has an unpaired electron making it highly reactive. It is produced as a result of radiolysis of water.

G

G1 The gap or growth period between telophase and the start of DNA synthesis when DNA is not replicating.

G2 The gap or growth period following the replication of DNA and prior to mitosis.

Gamete The mature male (spermatozoon) or female (ovum) reproductive cell.

Gene The basic unit of heredity that has a specific location on a chromosome.

Genetically significant dose (GSD) An average calculated from the gonadal dose received by the entire population and used to determine the genetic influence of low dose to the whole population.

Gonad shielding Protection of the reproductive organs from radiation exposure.

Gonadal dose A measure of the radiation to the patient at the site of the patient's gonads.

Granulocytes Red blood cells with a life cycle of one day.

H

Half-value layer (HVL) The thickness of the material that will reduce the X-ray intensity to half its original value.

Haploid Having half the diploid number of chromosomes found in somatic cells. Referred to as n; in humans, the n or haploid number = 23.

HeLa Letters that represent the first two letters of the patient's first and last names in an experiment conducted by Puck using uterine cervix cells to produce cell cultures.

Hemopoietic Pertaining to the development of blood cells.

Hypoxic Low levels of oxygen.

I

Image intensification fluoroscopy A procedure used to increase the brightness of an image with a decreased exposure time.

Indirect effect A cell interaction that occurs if the initial ionizing incident takes place on a distant noncritical molecule that then transfers the ionization of energy to another molecule.

Inflammation Redness and swelling at site of exposure.

Inherent filtration Limiting the X-ray beam by the use of a glass window in the tube and cooling oil surrounding the tube housing.

Intensifying screen A device that serves to accelerate the action of X-rays by converting X-ray energy into visible light.

Intermittent fluoroscopy The procedure of periodically activating the fluoroscopic tube rather than having the tube continuously activated; this reduces patient exposure and prolongs the life of the tube.

Interphase The period between cell divisions, known as the resting stage, when DNA is being synthesized. (Also known as S phase, S = synthesis.)

Interphase death Cell death occurring before mitosis.

Inverse square law The intensity of radiation at a given distance is inversely proportional to the square of the distance of the object from the source.

Involuntary motion Movement by the patient that is beyond his control.

Ionization chamber A tube containing a positive and negative electrode that are charged before use. One electrode is stationary; the other is moving. Exposure to ionization is determined by measuring the movement of the moving electrode.

J

Joint Commission The accrediting body for radiographic facilities.

K

Karyotype Chromosome map.

L

Late effect of radiation The response of human cells exposed to radiation months to years after exposure.

Latent The second stage in the response to radiation exposure in which changes are taking place within the body system that may either result in death or recovery.

Law of Bergonie and Tribondeau Law which states that ionizing radiation is more effective against cells that are highly mitotic, immature, and have a long dividing future; named for the two experimenters who made this determination.

LD50/30 The survival time of a specific group; the lethal dose to kill 50% of a population in 30 days.

LD50/60 The survival time of a specific group; the lethal dose to kill 50% of a population in 60 days.

Lead equivalent The amount of material that is needed to meet the same requirements as a lead barrier.

Lesion Open wound.

Leukemia Cancer of blood-forming cells in bone marrow.

Linear dose-response curve Graphical representation of relationship between radiation dose and observed response, in which any dose may have a potential effect, and there is a direct relationship between radiation dose and observed effect.

Linear energy transfer (LET) A measure of the rate at which energy is deposited from ionizing radiation to soft tissue.

Linear quadratic dose-response curve Graphical representation of relationship between radiation dose and observed response, in which the curve is linear or proportional at low doses, and becomes curvilinear at higher doses. This type of curve has no threshold.

Loci Spot, place of origin.

Lymphoid Lymph tissue.

M

Macromolecule A large molecule, for example, proteins, polymers, nucleic acids, and polysaccharides.

Malignant Progressive; threatening.

Manifest The third stage in the response to radiation exposure in which body systems show signs and symptoms of exposure.

Maturation depletion Reduction in the number of mature sperm.

Megakaryocytes Precursors for platelets.

Meiosis Cell division of germ cells, which consists of two cell divisions but only one replication of DNA. This results in each daughter cell containing one-half the number of chromosomes that is characteristic of the somatic cells of that species.

Meningitis Inflammation of the membranes of the spinal cord and brain.

Messenger RNA (m-RNA) RNA that binds amino acids to ribosomes during protein synthesis.

Metaphase The stage of mitosis where chromosomes are arranged.

Mitosis Type of cell division involving somatic cells in which a parent cell divides to create two daughter cells that contain the same chromosome number and DNA content as the parent. A continuous process having four phases: prophase, metaphase, anaphase, and telophase.

Mutagenesis The causing of genetic mutation by radiation.

Mutation A structural change or transformation of a chromosome that can be transmitted to offspring.

Myelocytes Precursors for white blood cells.

Myeloid Marrow.

N

Necrosis Tissue death.

Neoplasm Tumor.

Neuroblasts Embryonic nerve cells.

Nonstochastic Deterministic.

Nonthreshold Any dose received, regardless of size, that will produce a response.

Nuclear membrane Also referred to as the nuclear envelope; a two-layered membrane that surrounds the cell nucleus.

Nucleolus Spherical body in the cell nucleus that holds nuclear RNA. On the equatorial cell plane prior to separation, follows prophase and precedes anaphase.

O

Oogonia Reproductive cells of the female.

Optically stimulated luminescence (OSL) dosimeter A type of dosimeter utilizing aluminum oxide crystals to calculate the amount of personnel exposure.

Organism Any living entity; may be unicellular or multicellular.

Osteosarcoma Bone cancer.

Oxygen effect Name given to cellular response to radiation when oxygen is present.

P

Papillary Nipple-like, protruding.

Parenchymal Essential life-sustaining cells.

Personnel dosimeters Devices used to measure radiation doses.

Pocket dosimeter A type of dosimeter that uses an ionization chamber to determine the level of exposure by personnel.

Point mutation A mutation that occurs as a result of a change to a single DNA base pair, created by one nucleotide being exchanged for another.

Polymer A molecule created by combining two or more of the same molecules.

Primary protective barrier A fixed barrier that is located perpendicular to the line of travel of the primary X-ray beam.

Prodromal The first stage in the response to radiation exposure; nausea, vomiting, and diarrhea usually occur in this stage of exposure.

Progeny Offspring.

Prophase The first stage of mitosis or meiosis, when chromosomes become visible.

Protective tube housing The lead-lined metal covering of the X-ray beam that serves to reduce leakage radiation.

Protoplasm A colloidal structure of organic and inorganic materials and water that form the living cell.

R

Rad The unit of radiation absorbed dose.

Radiation cataractogenesis Formation of cataracts caused by exposure to radiation.

Radiation hormesis The controversial hypothesis that chronic low doses of ionizing radiation stimulates repair mechanisms that protect against disease.

Radiation protection Methods used to limit exposure to radiation.

Radioactivity The capability of a material to give off rays or particles from its nucleus.

Radiobiology Division of biology concerned with effects of ionizing radiation on living things.

Radiocarcinogenesis Radiation producing cancer.

Radiolysis Breakdown of water using radiation.

Radioresistant Having no reaction or ill effects of exposure to radiation.

Radiosensitivity The amount of reaction or response of a cell to radiation.

Radium Radiogenic substance.

Radon Radiogenic gas.

Relative biologic effectiveness (RBE) A comparison of how effective types of radiation are compared with X- and gamma-rays.

Relative risk model (1) Relates age at the time of radiation exposure to cancer risk estimate; also known as the multiplicative risk model. (2) The ratio of cancer incidence in an exposed population to that of an unexposed population.

Rem The unit of dose equivalent or occupational exposure.

Reproductive failure Cell that is unable to continue repeated divisions after being irradiated.

Ribonucleic acid (RNA) Nucleic acid that controls protein synthesis. Differs from DNA by having ribose as its sugar and the base uracil instead of thymine. Types include messenger, transfer, and ribosomal RNA.

Ribosomal RNA RNA that exists in ribosomes and assists in protein synthesis.

Ring Mutation of chromosome causing it to become ring-shaped.

Roentgen (R) A unit of radiation exposure descriptive of X- or gamma-radiation, the quantity of which would produce a charge of one electrostatic unit of electricity.

S

Scattered radiation Radiation that is dissipated away from the point of origin.

Sebaceous Oily secretion.

Secondary protective barrier A fixed barrier that is located parallel to the line of travel of the primary X-ray beam.

SED50 Radiation dose necessary to affect 50% of a population.

Shadow shield A radiopaque material that is suspended from the tube housing, which casts a shadow over the area that should not be exposed.

Shaped contact shield Lead devices that are shaped to fit over anatomical areas of the body to protect them from radiation exposure.

Sigmoid An S-shaped type of dose-response relationship.

Skin dose A measure of the radiation to the patient's skin at the skin entrance surface; also known as the entrance skin exposure (ESE).

Skin erythema dose (SED) A measure of the amount of radiation a person received.

Somatic Nonreproductive cells.

Source-image receptor distance (SID) The area from the point of contact on the patient to the tube.

Spermatogonia Reproductive cells of the male.

S-phase Period of synthesis or replication, the phase of the cell cycle after G1 and prior to G2.

Stem cell Immature cell.

Stochastic Occurring randomly in nature.

Stroma Supportive tissue of an organism.

Subcutaneous Inner layer of skin; the fatty layer.

Syndrome The relationship of signs and symptoms to a specific disease or trauma.

System A group of cells that perform a particular function.

T

Telophase The fourth or final stage of mitosis or meiosis, during which there is reconstruction of the nuclear membrane, and cell cytoplasm divides, giving birth to two daughter cells.

Thermoluminescent dosimeters (TLD) A type of dosimeter containing lithium fluoride or calcium fluoride crystals to calculate the amount of personnel exposure.

Threshold The point where a stimulus starts to produce an effect.

Threshold dose The dose at which symptoms will occur.

Time of occupancy (T) The amount of time a hospital area is occupied by people.

Total filtration The maximum amount of limitation of the X-ray beam through the use of both added and inherent filtration methods.

Transfer RNA (t-RNA) RNA that carries amino acids to ribosomes for assisting in protein synthesis.

Translocation Altering of a chromosome either by a portion of it transferring to another chromosome or to another section of the same chromosome.

Turner's syndrome An endocrine disorder caused by the failure of the ovaries to respond to pituitary hormone stimulation.

U

Uncontrolled area An area occupied by nonradiation personnel.

Use (U) The percentage of time in which the X-ray beam is energized and directed toward a particular wall.

Useful beam The primary X-ray beam.

V

Variable-aperture collimator A pair of upper- and lower-level lead shutters at right angles to each other. They can be adjusted to limit the field size the X-ray beam will expose.

Vasculitis Inflammation of blood vessels.

Voluntary motion Movement controlled by the patient.

W

Workload (W) The amount of activity of the X-ray machinery.

Z

Zygote Fertilized egg.

Index

CL

612.
014
48
FOR